DEJA REVIEW™

Psychiatry

Notice

Medicine is an ever-changing science. As new research and clinical experience broaden our knowledge, changes in treatment and drug therapy are required. The authors and the publisher of this work have checked with sources believed to be reliable in their efforts to provide information that is complete and generally in accord with the standards accepted at the time of publication. However, in view of the possibility of human error or changes in medical sciences, neither the authors nor the publisher nor any other party who has been involved in the preparation or publication of this work warrants that the information contained herein is in every respect accurate or complete, and they disclaim all responsibility for any errors or omissions or for the results obtained from use of the information contained in this work. Readers are encouraged to confirm the information contained herein with other sources. For example and in particular, readers are advised to check the product information sheet included in the package of each drug they plan to administer to be certain that the information contained in this work is accurate and that changes have not been made in the recommended dose or in the contraindications for administration. This recommendation is of particular importance in connection with new or infrequently used drugs.

DEJA REVIEW™

Psychiatry

Second Edition

Abilash A. Gopal, MD

Chief Resident, Department of Psychiatry
Langley Porter Psychiatric Institute
University of California, San Francisco
San Francisco, California

Alexander E. Ropper, MD

Resident Physician, Department of Neurosurgery
Brigham and Women's Hospital/Children's Hospital Boston
Harvard Medical School
Boston, Massachusetts

Louis A. Tramontozzi III, MD

Chief Resident, Department of Neurology
Tufts Medical Center
St. Elizabeth's Medical Center
Lahey Clinic Medical Center
Tufts University School of Medicine
Boston, Massachusetts

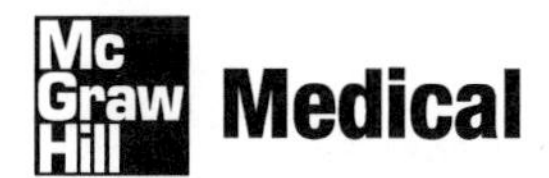

New York Chicago San Francisco Lisbon London Madrid Mexico City
Milan New Delhi San Juan Seoul Singapore Sydney Toronto

The McGraw·Hill Companies

Déjà Review™: Psychiatry, Second Edition

1 2 3 4 5 6 7 8 9 0 DOC/DOC 15 14 13 12 11

ISBN 978-0-07-171516-4
MHID 0-07-171516-9

This book was set in Palatino by Glyph International.

The editors were Kirsten Funk and Christine Diedrich.

The production supervisor was Catherine Saggese.

Project management was provided by Tania Andrabi, Glyph International.

RR Donnelley was printer and binder.

This book is printed on acid-free paper.

Library of Congress Cataloging-in-Publication Data

Gopal, Abilash A.
Deja review. Psychiatry / Abilash A. Gopal, Alexander E. Ropper, Louis A. Tramontozzi III.—2nd ed.
p. ; cm.—(Deja review) Psychiatry
Includes index.
ISBN-13: 978-0-07-171516-4 (pbk. : alk. paper)
ISBN-10: 0-07-171516-9 (pbk. : alk. paper) 1. Psychiatry—Examinations, questions, etc. I. Ropper, Alexander E. II. Tramontozzi, Louis A. III. Title. IV. Title: Psychiatry. V. Series: Deja review.
[DNLM: 1. Mental Disorders—Examination Questions. 2. Psychiatry—Examination Questions. WM 18.2]
RC457.G57 2011
616.890076—dc22

2011000447

Contents

Faculty Reviewer

Jason Yanofski, MD
Staff Psychiatrist
Traumatic Brain Injury
United States Army
Bamberg, Germany

Student Reviewers

Meredith Bergman
Fourth Year Medical Student
Weill-Cornell Medical College
Class of 2009

Michael S. Day
Third Year Medical Student
Weill-Cornell Medical College
Class of 2010

Brandon McKinney
Third Year Medical Student
University of Michigan
School of Medicine
Class of 2010

Lindsey Shultz
Fourth Year Medical Student
Weill-Cornell Medical College
Class of 2010

Acknowledgments

To all those who have opened our eyes to the great possibilities in medicine…

…and in particular, to those who have provided us with support, encouragement, and advice throughout this exciting project, such as Dr. Allan Ropper, Meghan Tramontozzi, and our respective families.

Preface

Déjà Review Psychiatry, Second Edition, was written with the intent to provide 3rd-year medical students with a comprehensive overview of the information they will encounter in their psychiatry clerkship. The information is presented using brief, bullet-point questions and answers in order to improve the usability of the text without sacrificing content. We attempted to draw students' attention to important and high-yield concepts by using boldface terms and stylized exclamation points. In addition, we encourage students to spend time learning the material presented at the end of each chapter consisting of clinical vignettes, which model the format of both the Boards and Psychiatry shelf exams.

ORGANIZATION

The *Deja Review* series is a unique resource that has been designed to allow you to review the essential facts and determine your level of knowledge on the subjects tested on your clerkship shelf exams, as well as the United States Medical Licensing Examination (USMLE) Step 2 CK. All concepts are presented in a question and answer format that covers key facts on commonly tested topics during the clerkship.

This question and answer format has several important advantages:

- It provides a rapid, straightforward way for you to assess your strengths and weaknesses.
- Prepares you for "pimping" on the wards.
- It allows you to efficiently review and commit to memory a large body of information.
- It serves as a quick, last-minute review of high-yield facts.
- Compact, condensed design of the book is conducive to studying on the go.

At the end of each the chapter, you will find clinical vignettes. These vignettes are meant to be representative of the types of questions tested on board and shelf exams to help you further evaluate your understanding of the material.

HOW TO USE THIS BOOK

This book is intended to serve as a tool during your psychiatry clerkship. Remember, this text is not intended to replace comprehensive textbooks, course packs, or lectures. It is simply intended to serve as a supplement to your studies during your psychiatry rotation and throughout your preparation for Step 2 CK. The previous edition was thoroughly reviewed by a number of medical students to represent the core topics tested on shelf examinations. For this reason, we encourage you to begin using this book early in your clinical years to reinforce topics you encounter while on the wards. You may use the book to quiz yourself or classmates on topics covered in recent lectures and clinical case discussions. A bookmark is included so that you can easily cover up the answers as you work through each chapter. The compact, condensed design of the book is conducive to studying on the go. Carry it in your white coat pocket so that you can access during any downtime throughout your busy day.

Our primary goals are that the text is easy-to-use, clear, and comprehensive. We invite students that use the book to send us suggestions for improvements to be incorporated into future editions.

Thanks for reading, and good luck on the wards!

Abilash A. Gopal, MD
Alexander E. Ropper, MD
Louis A. Tramontozzi III, MD

CHAPTER 1

Classic Psychology

! **What are the three main psychological theories that contribute most to psychotherapy?**	Psychoanalytic, cognitive, and behavioral

PSYCHOANALYTIC THEORY AND FREUD

What two concepts form the basis of Freud's theories on human behavior?	1. Unconscious motivations 2. Early developmental influences
! **What are the names and functions of Freud's three-part psychic structure of mind?**	1. *Id*—the mind's drives and instincts; these are always unconscious 2. *Ego*—resolves conflict and allows adaptation to one's environment 3. *Superego*—sense of right and wrong as created by parental and societal morality
What is the major function of the ego, and how does it accomplish this function?	The ego serves to reduce anxiety by employing a variety of defense mechanisms. Some of these mechanisms are considered to be more functional and mature than others.
! **What is a defense mechanism?**	An unconscious reaction employed by the ego in an attempt to decrease anxiety when confronted with feelings or ideas causing distress
How does an immature defense mechanism differ from a mature one?	Immature defense mechanisms distort reality to a greater degree than mature.

When are defense mechanisms pathologic?

- When they do not actually reduce anxiety
- When they prevent adaptation to a stressful situation
- When they decrease anxiety at the expense of increasing anxiety in the future

! **What are examples of mature defense mechanisms?**

SSIRAH for the mature wine drinkers

- *Somewhat mature:* **S**ublimation, **S**uppression, **I**ntellectualization, **R**ationalization
- *Most mature:* **A**ltruism, **H**umor

! **What are examples of immature defense mechanisms?**

DIaPeRS for the immature

DDD: **D**enial, **D**isplacement, **D**istortion

III: **I**dentification, **I**ntrojection, **I**solation

P: **P**rojection

RRR: **R**eaction formation, **R**egression, **R**epression

S: **S**omatization

! **What is sublimation?**

The conversion of unacceptable feelings or ideas into more acceptable actions. For example, a man is angry at his boss and unconsciously wishes to hurt him but instead he goes to the gym for an intense workout.

! **What is suppression?**

Avoiding distressing emotions or events while keeping them as components of conscious awareness by occupying oneself with other emotions or events. For example, a man who is having symptoms of a heart attack goes to the emergency room to be examined rather than be overwhelmed with fears about dying.

What is intellectualization?

Changing an emotionally disturbing problem into an entirely cognitive one. For example, a woman undergoing a divorce begins to read books about the legal and sociologic aspects of the process.

What is rationalization?

Distorting reality to make an undesirable event more palatable. For example, a student who is not elected to an honor society remarks that he is better off because he would have had to attend several meetings that would be wasteful of his time.

What is altruism?

Decreasing one's own anxiety or fears about a problem by helping or caring for others. For example, an obese woman lobbies for legislation to rid public schools of vending machines that sell soda.

What is humor?

Making light of one's own situation in an effort to decrease anxiety. For example, a bald man who is rejected on a date later tells bald jokes about himself to his friends.

! **What is denial?**

The unconscious refusal to acknowledge an event that allows a person to forget that such an event has occurred. For example, when asked by her new primary care physician, a breast cancer survivor says that she has no past medical problems.

! **What is displacement?**

Redirecting disturbing emotions about an object, idea, or event to a less threatening substitute. For example, a woman who was raped by a stranger complains that her husband does not respect her body.

What is distortion?

Altering one's perception of disturbing aspects of an external reality to make it more acceptable. For example, a motorist who is pulled over for running a stop sign explains that the stop sign was placed in an inconspicuous place.

What is identification?

Placing oneself in the shoes of another person who is perceivably more powerful or highly regarded. For example, in an effort to be promoted, an employee starts to carry a briefcase identical to that of his boss as well as wear a necktie while his coworkers do not.

What is introjection?

The absorption of qualities belonging to another person or object into one's own persona. For example, a shy teenager transfers to a high school where he joins the soccer team. He befriends the captain of the team and begins to act as he does: aggressively, loudly, and defiantly.

What is isolation?

Making a traumatic event more tolerable by separating the emotional experience from the physical event. For example, a survivor of the World Trade Center tragedy in New York City describes the cost and mechanics of tearing down the remaining steel structure without alluding to the emotional toll he has suffered.

! **What is projection?**

Taking distressing feelings, particularly anger and guilt, and attributing them to others. For example, a woman angry about burning her dinner accuses her roommate of being angry with her.

! **What is reaction formation?**

Converting an unacceptable or distressing emotion into its opposite. For example, a daughter angry at her mother for never being around when she was growing up visits her in the nursing home every week with fresh flowers.

What is regression?

Escaping back into an earlier developmental stage when confronted with a distressing event or feeling. For example, a patient who learns of her lung cancer diagnosis begins to skip around the halls of the hospital singing songs from her childhood.

What is repression?

Burying a distressing event or feeling into the unconscious to avoid or postpone confrontation. For example, a patient dying of emphysema is not aware that she will die despite what several doctors have told her.

! What is somatization?

The transference of an emotional distress into a physical manifestation. For example, a child angry that he has to eat vegetables claims that he has a stomachache.

What is the basis of drive psychology?

Freud believed that infants have pleasure-seeking drives and pass through specific stages of psychosexual development.

! What are the stages of psychosexual development?

In chronologic order, each stage describes the source of gratification for the individual:

1. *Oral*—first 18 months of life. The infant stimulates himself or herself by biting, sucking, or feeding. Excessive stimulation may lead to "oral fixation" and problems of dependency later in life.
2. *Anal*—between 18 and 36 months. As the child is struggling to exert autonomy, he or she seeks pleasure in controlling the passage of stool, receiving stimulation from holding it in or letting it out. Overly strict or inconsistent toilet training may result in the acquirement of "anal traits" such as stubbornness or inflexibility as seen in obsessive-compulsive personality.
3. *Phallic*—begins at 3 years of life. The child discovers his own penis or her own clitoris as a source of pleasure. There is a transition in the search for gratification from one's body to an external source.
   - *Oedipal*—between 3 and 5 years of age and resultant from the search in the phallic stage. Boys compete with their fathers as they struggle with their erotic love for their own mother. Resolution of this struggle ends in identification with their father and transference of love to other women. Girls struggle similarly with erotic love for their father and competition with their mother. (Later referred to as the Electra Complex by Jung.)

4. *Latency*—between 5 and 11-13 years of age. Psychosexual development takes a back seat to more pressing tasks at hand such as developing relationships with peers and acquiring necessary skills.
5. *Genital*—begins with puberty and ends in young adulthood. This marks a momentous return of psychosexual development as the adolescent begins to relate to peers in a sexual way in the journey toward a suitable partner and away from parental figures.

COGNITIVE THEORY

! **What is the focus of cognitive theory?**

Cognitive theory focuses on *how* the individual experiences events rather than the events themselves.

What is a schema or cognitive framework?

A certain way of thinking about oneself, others, or the world. Adopting a particular schema determines how a person will feel about an event.

! **According to cognitive theory, how do schemas lead to psychopathology?**

- A pattern of behavior develops based on faulty schemas.
- Faulty schemas arise from previous negative experiences and are distorted by irrational beliefs.
- These schemas are reinforced through the powerful emotions they elicit.
- When an individual attributes an irrational emotion to a particular event, he or she may suffer from its psychological or physical consequences.

! **What are some examples of cognitive distortions?**

1. *Arbitrary inference:* coming to a conclusion without adequate evidence
2. *Dichotomous thinking:* classifying an experience as one extreme or the other
3. *Overgeneralization:* making a general conclusion on the basis of one event
4. *Magnification:* making too much out of a bad thing

5. *Minimization:* making too little out of a good thing
6. *Selective abstraction:* focusing on one negative aspect to make a conclusion while ignoring the positive aspects
7. *Personalization:* incorrectly or inappropriately attributing external events to oneself

BEHAVIORAL THEORY

What is the basis of behavioral theory?

Behaviors are learned from the environment or through reward.

What is modeling?

The observation and replication of someone else's behavior.

What is classical conditioning?

Learning to behave in a certain way in response to a neutral stimulus in the environment. (Remember Pavlov's dogs who salivated at the sound of a bell even in the absence of food after a period of hearing the bell with each meal.)

! **What is operant conditioning?**

Learning to behave in such a way that will result in a reward or will avoid a punishment.

What is "temperament"?

The idea that infants are born with an inherited set of traits governing how they react to the environment and what they require for care. These traits are stable for the first few years of life but outside forces may modulate them.

What are the three types of temperament?

Easy, difficult, and slow to warm up. These types describe how children respond to change, their sleeping and eating habits, mood, and emotional reactions.

TYPES OF PSYCHOTHERAPY

! **What is behavioral psychotherapy?**	Attempting to reshape an individual's behavior and extinguish maladaptive behaviors without addressing his or her inner conflicts
What is brief individual psychotherapy?	A short course of therapy spread over a predetermined number of meetings focused on a troubling aspect in a persons life and not his or her overall psychiatric makeup
In cognitive therapy, how does "cognitive restructuring" work?	The therapist helps the patient to find ways of correcting negative schemas by creating healthier, more adaptive ways of thinking. Together they will identify the patient's erroneous beliefs and prove their irrationality by citing contradictory objective evidence from other aspects of the patient's life.
! **What is cognitive-behavioral psychotherapy?**	Use of cognitive and behavioral theories to change the way patients think about themselves, others, or the world and subsequently change the patterns of behavior they learned from these schemas. This is usually a short-term therapy.
What is family therapy?	Identification of problems in the dynamics of how a family functions and modifying interactions within this unit to promote change and improve functioning
! **What is group therapy?**	An individual finds therapeutic gain both through hearing the experiences and coping strategies shared by other members of a group and by contributing to the group.

! **What is psychodynamic psychotherapy?**

The use of psychodynamic theory to facilitate a patient's understanding of how previous experiences as early as childhood, some even relegated to the unconscious, contribute to a current state of psychopathology. Techniques used by the therapist include listening, asking questions, encouraging free associations, recollection of emotionally significant events, and discussion of transference and defenses.

! **What is transference?**

The projection of feelings, thoughts, and wishes onto the psychoanalyst who comes to represent someone from the patient's past

What is countertransference?

The analyst's projection of his or her own emotional needs and desires onto the patient

What is dialectical behavior therapy?

A system of therapy originally developed to treat persons with borderline personality disorder (BPD) by Marsha M. Linehan. BDP combines standard cognitive-behavioral techniques for emotion regulation with concepts of distress tolerance, acceptance, and mindful awareness largely derived from Buddhist meditative practice.

What is the goal of dialectical behavior therapy?

To reduce suicidal gestures in patients suffering from borderline personality disorder

! **What is supportive psychotherapy?**

The essential component of supportive therapy is to "support" the individual's defenses using validation, empathy, education, and reality testing. A therapeutic relationship is formed with the patient by encouraging him or her to express the emotions without being judgmental. Several psychotherapies incorporate an aspect of supportive psychotherapy.

CLINICAL VIGNETTES

A 14-year-old boy asks his parents if they need their cars washed. The cars are not particularly dirty, and he washed them only 5 days ago. The boy has never seemed this eager to do chores around the house. About 2 months ago his father gave him $20 to wash his car. According to behavioral theory, what type of conditioning has affected this boy?

Operant conditioning; behavioral theory proposes that behaviors are learned from the environment or through reward. This boy's behavior can be explained by operant conditioning. He has learned that washing his parents' cars will result in a monetary reward so he seeks out this behavior. Another example of operant conditioning is behavior learned to avoid a punishment. Operant conditioning should not be confused with classical conditioning, which describes behavior learned by responding to a neutral stimulus in the environment.

A 43-year-old woman follows up with her psychiatrist for anxiety and depression. Although she receives pharmacologic therapy, she feels that she also benefits from psychotherapy. She has been seeing this psychiatrist for 2 years now on a regular basis. During her visits she does most of the talking, and the psychiatrist mainly listens to her. Over the years she has talked much about her childhood conflicts with her mother. The psychiatrist has encouraged her to remember emotionally significant events during this stage of her life as he believes they have great significance on her present day problems. She has come to the realization that her anxiety comes from the pressure of high expectations put on her by her mother. She also now believes that her conflicting thoughts about her father have contributed to her depression. What type of therapy has this psychiatrist used with his patient?

Psychodynamic psychotherapy; in this form of therapy the psychiatrist uses psychodynamic theory to facilitate a patient's understanding of how previous experiences as early as childhood, some even relegated to the unconscious, contribute to a current state of psychopathology. Techniques used by the therapist include listening, asking questions, encouraging free associations and recollection of emotionally significant events, and discussing transference and defenses.

A 46-year-old man follows up with his psychiatrist for depression. He has been taking a selective serotonin reuptake inhibitor (SSRI) for 2 years now with good results. Initially his sleep patterns were disturbed, feelings of guilt persisted, decreased energy and lack of initiative prevented him from being successful at work, and his mood was generally low. In addition to pharmacologic treatment this patient has agreed to participate in psychotherapy. With his psychiatrist the patient has identified how he thinks about the outside world. He believes his coworkers have little faith in his ability and that his family feels that he is a failure. He makes a list of events at work and at home that contradict his beliefs. Making this list helps him to realize that his beliefs are in fact erroneous. What type of therapy is this psychiatrist using and what specific technique has been employed with this patient?

Cognitive restructuring in cognitive therapy; this psychiatrist has used cognitive therapy to help the patient find ways of correcting negative schemas by creating healthier, more adaptive ways of thinking. By employing the technique of cognitive restructuring, the psychiatrist assists his patient in making a list of factual events to prove that his beliefs are irrational and erroneous. This patient realizes that his coworkers must have faith in his work if he recently received a commendation. He also realizes that his family recognizes his success since they acknowledge his accomplishments.

A 43-year-old woman has been homeless for 5 years since her husband left her and she lost her job. She lived on the street and moved from one shelter to another. Through one of the job skills training programs at a shelter she learned how to sew and obtained a job at a tailor's shop where she has worked for 8 months now. She saved enough money to move into a small apartment where she pays monthly rent. She remembers what it was like to be homeless and fears that something bad will happen to her that will cause her to lose her apartment so that she will be homeless again. Three nights each week she volunteers at the homeless shelter giving out food and helping to teach job skills. What defense mechanism has this woman employed?

Altruism; she has demonstrated altruism by finding a way to help or care for other people so as to decrease her own anxiety or fears about becoming homeless again. Altruism is a mature defense mechanism learned during late childhood or early adulthood and distorts external reality to a lesser degree than an immature defense mechanism.

A 4-year-old boy spends most of his day with his mother. He goes to preschool for a couple of hours each day but always spends the rest of the day with his mother. They go shopping together, eat their meals together, and play together. He has a sister who attends elementary school, and his father works as a lawyer. Around dinnertime his father comes home, embraces his wife, and kisses her in front of the children. The boy becomes enraged, crying, and tugging at his mother's pant leg. According to Freud, what stage of psychosexual development best characterizes the young boy?

Oedipal component of the phallic stage; Freud believed that infants have sexual drives and pass through specific stages of psychosexual development. In each stage the individual finds a different source of gratification. In this scenario, the boy is competing with his father for the love and attention of his mother. Freud believed this represented the infant's struggle with his erotic love for his own mother. This describes the oedipal component of the phallic stage of psychosexual development. Resolution of this struggle ends in identification with his father and transference of love to other women. The other stages of psychosexual development are oral, anal, latency, and genital.

A 53-year-old man is constantly belittled by his boss at his banking job. The boss is very critical of the man's job performance in front of his other coworkers. According to his boss, nothing ever seems to be done correctly when this man is responsible for a task. The boss has even started poking fun at the man's personal character in the office. Never before in previous jobs has this man been treated by a superior this way. He often feels humiliated and angry when he comes to work. For the boss's birthday the man gives him a birthday card and a generous gift certificate to his favorite restaurant. What defense mechanism has this man employed?

Reaction formation; he has demonstrated reaction formation by converting an unacceptable or distressing emotion into its opposite. Reaction formation is an immature defense mechanism learned during childhood and distorts an individual's external reality in an attempt to cope with a stressor. This defense mechanism is considered to be immature because it does not provide an effective means for adaptation. In this instance, the man's behavior does not address the actual source of anxiety; instead, he rewards his boss and most likely will continue to be belittled and treated poorly in the future.

A 40-year-old woman presents to the ER after slashing her wrists. This is the fifth time in her life that she has made a suicidal gesture, and she explains that death would be a way for her to escape the "emptiness" that plagues her. Her medical records indicate that she has seen many psychiatrists in the past. When asked why she has changed psychiatrists so many times, she states that they abandoned her and that it was not her fault. She goes on to comment that the doctors in the ER have treated her "perfectly," while the nursing staff has been "the worst" she has ever seen. What defense mechanism does this patient display? What treatment would be most effective for her illness?

Splitting. Treat with psychotherapy; the patient uses "splitting," a complex defense mechanism in which others are seen as either all good (and thus caring, rescuing sources of strength) or all bad (and thus to blame for all one's own misery). She suffers from borderline personality disorder, which involves a pervasive pattern of impulsivity and unstable relationships, affects self-image and behaviors, present by early adulthood and in a variety of contexts. The treatment of choice is psychotherapy.

A 62-year-old Irish-American woman plans a trip to Ireland with her husband. Because of her lower socioeconomic background, she had never previously traveled abroad. In fact she had never flown on an airplane before. She grew up in an Irish section of Boston close enough to the airport to see planes leaving and landing, and she would often imagine where they were going to or coming from. She prepared for her trip to Ireland for weeks and on the day of departure she and her husband were excited to go to the airport. When she presented her ticket at the counter she was told that her flight was delayed for 2 hours. This made her very upset, and she could not understand why the plane could not take off at the time it was scheduled. After returning from her trip she told her friends and coworkers that flights to Ireland are always delayed. What example of cognitive distortion has this woman employed?

Overgeneralization; making a general conclusion on the basis of one event characterizes the cognitive distortion of overgeneralization. Cognitive theory attributes importance not to the objective events that occur in one's life, but *how* the individual experiences these events.

CHAPTER 2

Mood Disorders

INTRODUCTION

What is mood?

A description of one's internal emotional state

What constitutes a mood disorder?

An abnormal range of moods associated with a loss of control over them

What is affect?

An assessment of how the patient's mood appears to the examiner

What dimensions are used to describe affect?

- *Quality*—depth/range of feeling. Flat (none) < blunted (shallow) < constricted (limited) < full (average) < intense (more than normal). A person with flat affect remains expressionless and monotone even when discussing happy or sad events.
- *Motility*—speed at which person shifts emotional states. Sluggish < supple < labile. A patient with labile affect might laugh one minute and cry the next.
- *Appropriateness*—whether affect is congruent with circumstances. Appropriate or inappropriate ("mood incongruent"). A person with inappropriate affect might giggle when describing a loved one's death.

MAJOR DEPRESSIVE DISORDER

Epidemiology and Etiology

What gender and age group are most at risk for developing major depressive disorder (MDD)?	Female to male ratio is 2:1. Highest risk from age 20 to 40
! What is the lifetime prevalence of MDD?	15%
What ethnicity and socioeconomic groups are most at risk for depression?	None. All are equally affected.
What is the concordance rate of depression in monozygotic and dizygotic twins?	50%-70% in monozygotic and 20% in dizygotic
! What is the risk of completed suicide in major depression?	15% over the course of a patient's lifetime
Abnormal levels of what neurotransmitter are believed to contribute to depression?	Serotonin
Dysfunction of what neuroendocrine axis is thought to be involved in depression?	Hypothalamic-pituitary-adrenal axis
How does behavioral theory explain depression?	"Learned helplessness": Depression results from repeated life experiences that lead to the belief that one can do little to improve his or her state of suffering or place in life.
How does cognitive theory explain depression?	"Faulty cognitive frameworks": Depression results from distorted, unrealistic, and unhelpful interpretations of one's environment.
How does psychodynamic theory explain depression?	The inability to adequately recover from the loss of relationships or attachment to something valuable
! What medications are thought to trigger depressive symptoms?	**Beta-blockers, corticosteroids,** benzodiazepines, and interferon

! What are some common medical causes of depressive symptoms?

Endocrine (**hypothyroidism**, adrenal dysfunction), neurologic (Parkinson disease, strokes, dementia), metabolic disorders (vitamin B_{12} deficiency), cancer (pancreatic), and infections (human immunodeficiency virus [HIV], hepatitis)

Diagnosis

! What are the *DSM-IV* (*Diagnostic and Statistical Manual of Mental Disorders, Fourth Edition*) criteria for diagnosing MDD?

Criteria for a major depressive episode requires five or more of the following symptoms to be present for at least 2 weeks as well as depressed mood or anhedonia: **SIGECAPS**

Sleep changes
Decreased **I**nterest
Guilt
Low **E**nergy
Decreased **C**oncentration
Appetite changes
Psychomotor agitation or retardation
Suicidality

Symptoms cannot be due to substance use or medical condition. They must cause social/occupational impairment.

What is anhedonia?

Loss of interest in normally pleasurable activities

How can depression present differently in the elderly population?

Elderly patients may complain of anxiety, irritability, weakness, difficulty concentrating, memory problems, or multiple somatic complaints such as headache, backache, gastrointestinal complaints, dizziness, numbness, fatigue, or lethargy.

What is the differential diagnosis of major depression?

Mood disorder because of general medical condition, substance-induced mood disorder, dysthymic disorder, bipolar disorder (BD), dementia, adjustment disorder with depressed mood, schizoaffective disorder and other psychotic disorders, and bereavement

What are some predisposing factors to major depression?

Chronic physical illness, alcohol and drug dependence, psychosocial stressors, female gender, family history of depression, prior depressive episodes, and childbirth

! What sleep disturbances are seen in depression?

Deep sleep (delta sleep, stages 3 and 4) is decreased in depression. Time spent in rapid eye movement (REM) sleep is increased and the onset of REM in the sleep cycle is earlier (decreased latency to REM). Some people report intermittent and **early morning awakenings**.

! What is the typical course of a depressive episode?

Depressive episodes last about 6-9 months if left untreated. Fifty percent of individuals who develop a single depressive episode will have additional episodes. The majority of those who suffer from a second episode will subsequently have a third.

What subtypes of depression exist?

- *Melancholic:* anhedonia, early morning awakenings, psychomotor disturbance, excessive guilt, and anorexia; 40%-60% of hospitalized patients with depression
- *Atypical:* hypersomnia, hyperphagia, reactive mood, leaden paralysis, and hypersensitivity to interpersonal rejection
- *Catatonic:* purposeless motor activity, extreme negativism or mutism, bizarre postures, and echolalia. Can also be applied to BD
- *Psychotic:* presence of hallucinations or delusions; 10%-25% of hospitalized patients with depression

These subtypes can be used to describe a patient's diagnosis, for example, "MDD with psychotic features."

What is seasonal affective disorder?

Subtype of depression that only occurs during winter months. Patients respond to treatment with light therapy.

Treatment (*see Chapter 14 for more detailed information on treatment*)

What are the main classes of antidepressants used to treat depression?

Selective serotonin reuptake inhibitors (SSRIs), tricyclic antidepressants (TCAs), monoamine oxidase inhibitors (MAOIs), selective noradrenaline reuptake inhibitors (SNRIs), and dopamine reuptake inhibitors

What are the different types of psychotherapy used to treat depression?

Cognitive-behavioral, supportive, brief interpersonal, and psychodynamic psychotherapies have the most data to support their efficacy in treating depression.

What are indications for using electroconvulsive therapy (ECT)?

- Depression refractory to antidepressants
- Contraindication to antidepressant medications
- Immediate risk for suicide
- History of good response to ECT
- Depression with psychotic features
- Pregnancy (may be safer than alternate treatments)

What are contraindications to using ECT?

- Recent cardiovascular event (eg, MI w/in last 6 months)
- Space-occupying brain lesions
- Increased intracranial pressure

How is ECT performed?

ECT is performed under general anesthesia with the aid of muscle relaxants. A seizure is induced by passing an electric current through the brain. The seizure lasts <1 minute. Approximately eight treatments are administered over a 2- to 3-week period, with significant improvement typically seen after the first week.

What are the major side effects associated with ECT?

- **Transient cognitive side effects** including confusion.
- **Anterograde amnesia** occurring during the course of ECT, disappearing days to weeks after completion of treatment. Most common amnesia seen in ECT
- **Retrograde amnesia**, which usually disappears after 6 months

How can side effects from ECT be minimized?

- Reducing the frequency of treatment from 3 to 2 times/week.
- Use of brief pulse rather than sine wave ECT machines.
- Unilateral or bifrontal positions of the electrodes instead of bitemporal.

Unfortunately, these techniques are also associated with less effective treatment of depression.

! How effective are the various treatment modalities for depression?

- Antidepressants alone achieve remission in 30%-50% of patients with up to 70% showing improvement.
- Combined treatment with psychotherapy and antidepressants achieves remission in 60%-70% of patients.
- ECT achieves remission in >75% of patients.

! What is the pharmacologic treatment regimen for a major depressive episode?

Antidepressants should be continued for at least 6 months and more often 8-12 months before a taper is initiated, during which time patients must be observed for signs of relapse. Patients may need to remain on antidepressants for longer if they have experienced several depressive episodes in the past or if they have a strong family history of depression.

BIPOLAR I DISORDER

Epidemiology and Etiology

What is the lifetime prevalence of bipolar I disorder (BD I)?

1%

Are there any gender disparities in the incidence of BD I?

No. Men and women are equally affected.

What is the typical age of onset of BD?

15-30 years

Is there a difference in age of onset of BD by gender?

Recent data suggest a 3-5 year earlier age of onset for men.

Is there a genetic predisposition to BD?

Yes: 40% concordance among monozygotic twins. First-degree relatives of BD patients have a 25% risk of any mood disorder.

! **What is the mortality rate in BD?**

10%-15% mortality by suicide

! **What are some risk factors for suicide completion?**

SAD PERSONS

Sex (male)
Age (**elderly** or **adolescent**)
Depression
Previous suicide attempts
Ethanol abuse
Rational thinking loss (psychosis)
Social support lacking
Organized plan to commit suicide
No spouse (divorced > widowed > single)
Sickness (physical illness)

Diagnosis

! **What are the diagnostic features of BD I?**

The occurrence of one manic or mixed episode. Between manic episodes, there may be euthymia, MDD, or hypomania, but none of these are required for the diagnosis.

What is a bipolar mixed episode (aka mixed mania or "dysphoric mania" state)?

Criteria are met for both mania and major depression nearly every day during at least a 1-week period. Increased energy and some form of anger, from irritability to full blown rage, are the most common symptoms. Symptoms may also include auditory hallucinations, confusion, insomnia, persecutory delusions, racing thoughts, restlessness, and suicidal ideation

! What are the characteristics of a manic episode as defined by the *DSM-IV*?

A period of abnormally and persistently elevated, expansive, or irritable mood, lasting at least 1 week and including at least three of the following: **DIG FAST**

Distractibility
Insomnia—decreased need for sleep
Grandiosity—inflated self-esteem
Flight of ideas or racing thoughts
Agitation or increase in goal-directed activity socially, at work, or sexually
Speech—pressured

Thoughtlessness—excessive involvement in pleasurable activities such as unrestrained shopping or high-risk sexual activity

Symptoms cannot be due to substance use or medical conditions.

Symptoms must cause social/occupational impairment.

What distinguishes mania from hypomania?

Duration and severity

- *Mania*—abnormal mood for at least 1 week unless hospitalization is required; symptoms severe enough to impair social/occupational functioning or presence of psychotic symptoms
- *Hypomania*—abnormal mood for at least 4 days; symptoms do not significantly impair ability to function (ie, milder symptoms)

What is the differential diagnosis of BD?

Other mood disorders, psychotic disorders with mood symptoms, mood disorder due to a general medical condition, and substance-induced mood disorder

What are some common medical causes of manic symptoms?

Endocrine (hyperthyroidism), neurologic (seizures, stroke), and systemic disorders (HIV, vitamin B_{12} deficiency)

! What medications/drugs tend to produce manic symptoms?

Stimulants (methylphenidate, dextroamphetamine), steroids, sympathomimetics, and antidepressants. Recreational drugs including cocaine, amphetamines, and alcohol. Withdrawal from alcohol or other central nervous system (CNS) depressants such as barbiturates and benzodiazepines can produce manic symptoms.

What is the typical course of a manic episode?	Mania develops over days and lasts about 3 months if untreated. More than 90% of patients will have a recurrence of their manic symptoms. Episodes may occur more frequently as the disease progresses.
What is meant by "rapid-cycling" BD?	Four or more mood disturbances (MDD, mania, or mixed) in 1 year
! **What are some known precipitants of manic episodes?**	Changes in sleep-wake cycle, **antidepressant treatmen**t, stressful life-events, and the postpartum period

Treatment (*see Chapter 14 for more detailed information on treatment*)

What are the medications used to treat mania?	**Lithium,** anticonvulsants (eg, **valproate [Depacon]** or **carbamazepine [Tegretol]),** and **antipsychotics** (eg, olanzapine [Zyprexa], risperidone [Risperdal], quetiapine [Seroquel], ziprasidone [Geodon], and aripiprazole [Abilify]). Benzodiazepines can be used adjunctively in acute mania for sedation. In severe cases, more than one class of medication (eg, lithium combined with an atypical antipsychotic and a benzodiazepine) may be used.
What are the medications commonly used to treat the depressive phase of BD I?	Lithium, Symbax (combination of olanzapine and fluoxetine), quetiapine (Seroquel), and lamotrigine (Lamictal). Given their potential to induce mania, antidepressants should be used with caution.
What medications are most often used to prevent recurrence of mood episodes (ie, maintenance therapy)?	Lithium, valproate (Depakote), atypical antipsychotics (eg, aripiprazole [Abilify] or olanzapine [Zyprexa]), and lamotrigine (Lamictal)
What medication is thought to be most effective in treating rapid-cycling BD?	There is some evidence that valproate (Depakote) may be most effective.
What adjunct therapies can be useful for patients with BD?	Supportive psychotherapy, family therapy, and group therapy
What nonpharmacologic treatment can be used for acute mania?	ECT

BIPOLAR II DISORDER

What is the lifetime prevalence of bipolar II disorder (BD II)?	0.5%
Are there any gender disparities in the incidence of BD II?	More common in women
! **What are the diagnostic features of BD II?**	History of one or more major depressive episodes and at least one hypomanic episode
In relation to depressive episodes, when do hypomanic episodes tend to occur?	Just prior to or following a depressive episode
What is the course of BD II?	Similar to BD I: tends to be chronic, requiring long-term treatment
What are the treatment goals and methods for BD II?	Same as BD I
! **What disorder is often different to distinguish from BD II?**	Borderline personality disorder (BPD). Both BPD and BD II involve "mood swings."
! **How does one distinguish between BD II and BPD?**	In BD II, mood episodes (hypomania and depression) generally last weeks or months. In BPD, there is marked mood lability ("emotional dysregulation") in response to external stressors, causing changes in mood lasting seconds, hours, or days.

OTHER MOOD DISORDERS

Epidemiology and Etiology

What is dysthymic disorder?	A mild, chronic form of major depression
What is the lifetime prevalence of dysthymia?	6%
What is the point prevalence of dysthymia?	3%

What age group is most at risk for developing dysthymia?

Patients younger than 25, although women aged 65 or younger are also at increased risk.

Are there any gender disparities in the incidence of dysthymia?

Yes. It is two to three times more common in women.

What percentage of patients with dysthymia will develop BD or major depression?

Less than 5% will develop BD I, and 20% will develop MDD.

What is the endocrine disorder most commonly associated with depressive symptoms?

Hypothyroidism

What type of cancers can manifest with depressive symptoms?

Pancreatic and oropharyngeal carcinomas

What is cyclothymic disorder?

Chronic fluctuating episodes of mild depression and hypomania, lasting a variable amount of time

What is the lifetime prevalence of cyclothymia?

Less than 1%

What age group is most at risk for cyclothymia?

Young adults (aged 15-25)

Diagnosis

! **What are the *DSM-IV* criteria for diagnosing dysthymia?**

Chronically depressed mood most of the time for a minimum of **2 years**

- At least **2** of the following:
  - Poor concentration
  - Hopelessness
  - Change in appetite
  - Change in sleep
  - Fatigue
  - Low self-esteem
- During the **2**-year period
  - No symptom-free period >**2** months
  - No major depressive episode

Think of the Rule of 2s: (2 y, ≥ 2 symptoms, no symptom-free period >2 mo)

What is meant by the term "double depression"?

Major depressive episodes occurring in conjunction with dysthymia

What is the differential diagnosis for dysthymia?

Major depression, mood disorder due to a general medical condition, and substance-induced mood disorder

! **What are the *DSM-IV* diagnostic criteria for cyclothymic disorder?**

- Numerous periods with hypomanic symptoms and periods with depressive symptoms for at least 2 years
- No symptom-free period >2 months during those 2 years
- No history of major depressive episode or manic episode

What diagnostic criteria differentiate cyclothymic disorder from BD II?

Chronic course and lack of a major depressive episode

A mood disorder with marked motor immobility, excessive and purposeless movement, or mutism is generally classified as what type of depression?

Catatonic depression

! **What is postpartum depression?**

Depression occurring within 4 weeks of delivery

What is melancholic depression?

Depression with severe vegetative features and profound feelings of guilt or remorse

! **Do all depressive episodes feature lack of sleep and weight loss?**

No. Patients with atypical depression may be hypersomnic, gain weight, and have excessive mood lability.

! **How long after the onset of substance use do mood disorder symptoms appear in a substance-induced mood disorder?**

Within 1 month of substance intoxication or withdrawal

Treatment

What is the most effective treatment for dysthymia?

Therapy (psychotherapy or cognitive therapy) in conjunction with antidepressant medications

How is cyclothymia usually treated?

Antimanic medications (eg, lithium, anticonvulsants, and antipsychotics) are generally used. It must be noted that patients diagnosed with this disorder are less likely to seek medical attention than patients with traditional mania or MDD.

What is the treatment for patients with substance-induced mood disorders?

Cessation of use of the drug or substance

If symptoms of a substance-induced mood disorder do not resolve within a few weeks after cessation of the causative substance, what is the best approach to treatment?

At this point, patients may benefit from an appropriately prescribed medication. It is important to treat the substance-abuse problems as well as the mood disorder.

CLINICAL VIGNETTES

A 26-year-old man has been extremely complimentary to his coworkers for the past week. He has purchased gifts for everyone at his office for no apparent reason. When asked how he had the time to buy and wrap each individual gift after working every day, he claims that he just "feels more energy" despite his surprising lack of sleep recently. His coworkers are confused when his mood completely changes a month later and he becomes avoidant, lethargic, and uninterested in his normal activities. He is overheard telling his boss that he feels as if life is not worth living anymore. What is the diagnosis?

Bipolar disorder (BD) II; this young man exhibits a major depressive episode which is preceded by an episode of hypomania. Although BD II has a more stable course and better prognosis when compared to BD I, the treatment is the same.

A 36-year-old woman is brought to the clinic by her husband because he is concerned about her "mood swings." He describes a 2-week period over the summer when she was very irritable and went on several shopping sprees, eventually reaching the limits on their credit card. Then, during winter holidays she would not leave the house. At the time she was tearful and unable to finish daily chores, complaining of a lack of energy and an inability to concentrate. This sort of episode happened again at the end of February. Recently, she has been staying up late and her husband is surprised at how much of a "go-getter" she has become. What is the diagnosis and how should she be treated?

Rapid-cycling BD. Treat with anticonvulsants for mood stabilization; because of the existence of four mood disturbances (in this case, two depressive and two manic) in 1 year, the diagnosis of rapid-cycling BD can be made. Stressful life events, disturbances in sleep-wake cycles, and the postpartum period can be triggers of mood disturbances in rapid-cycling BD. Valproate (Depacon) is thought to be more effective in treating rapid-cycling BD, but lithium is also first-line.

A 23-year-old woman reports difficulty concentrating at work. She says that she has suffered from inattentiveness for as long as she can remember and that she has "always" had a lack of energy and "never" seemed to find any activity that made her happy or excited. She denies any psychomotor or neurovegetative symptoms. What is the likely diagnosis?

Dysthymia; since this patient is presenting with a history of chronic, mild depression the most likely diagnosis is dysthymia. Given this history, the criteria for a major depressive disorder are not met.

A 28-year-old man complains to his primary care physician who recently started treating his hypertension that he is not sleeping well, has lost interest in playing in his corporate softball league, and feels "down." His vitals are T 98.6°F, HR 78, BP 128/82, and RR 14. What diagnosis must the physician rule out?

Substance-induced mood disorder; the patient may be taking a beta-blocker for his hypertension, which can induce depressive symptoms.

A 78-year-old man is brought to the psychiatrist by his daughter because he has been sad recently. His wife died 2 months ago from breast cancer after 48 years of marriage. The man is neatly dressed and admits to thinking about his wife often. He complains of "not sleeping well or eating much." He has continued to volunteer at the local soup kitchen as he has since retirement. What information must the psychiatrist elicit when making the diagnosis of depression in the context of grief?

Duration of symptoms, functionality, and presence of psychotic symptoms or suicidal ideation; there is much variation in what different individuals and cultural groups deem "normal bereavement." Functional impairment, suicidal ideation, psychomotor agitation, severe or unrealistic guilt, marked hallucinations and delusions, and symptoms that persist for more than 2 months are abnormal reactions to grief and may point to a diagnosis of depression.

A 26-year-old woman gave birth to a healthy baby boy 3 weeks ago. Her husband has noticed that she doubts her ability to care for the child and that she is crying on a daily basis. She has not had any thoughts of harming herself or the child. What is the diagnosis, and what is its prevalence?

Postpartum depression, prevalence of 10-15% in new mothers; the same criteria for depression are used to diagnosis postpartum depression, which should be distinguished from postpartum "blues," a mild dysphoric illness that occurs in up to 50% of postpartum women.

An 18-year-old college freshman has not slept for 4 days because he has felt "full of energy." He successfully finished an exam in one of his classes on Friday and attended his morning classes on Monday without any difficulty. Over the weekend and through Tuesday he socialized with numerous friend groups, and his friends noted his mood to be elevated. What is the diagnosis?

Hypomania; despite this man's abnormal mood for 4 days, he was still able to take an exam, socialize, and attend classes. With at least 4 days of abnormal mood and without significant impairment of functioning, a diagnosis of hypomania can be made and should be differentiated from mania.

A 53-year-old mother of three with no past medical history complains that over the last 5 days she has experienced decreased concentration, feelings of guilt, trouble sleeping, and low energy. She also says that she skipped her book club meeting yesterday because she did not think it would be any fun. What is the diagnosis?

Depressive disorder not otherwise specified; the diagnosis of major depressive disorder cannot be made until the criteria for depression are present for at least 2 weeks. The diagnosis "depressive disorder not otherwise specified" may be appropriate for presentations of depressed mood with clinically significant impairment that do not meet criteria for duration or severity.

A 19-year-old presents to the ER accompanied by the coach of his football team. He seems animated and claims that he is "ready to play in the NFL." His coach notes that although he has not been sleeping much in the previous week, he has seemed full of energy. During the interview, the teenager begins making sexual advances on a nurse in the room and eventually must be restrained by three security guards. The physician on duty contacts the boy's father, who states that the boy has no history of this sort of behavior. On admission to the hospital, the boy states that he is ready to use his "healing magic" on other patients. What is the most likely diagnosis? What is the treatment of choice?

BD I. Treatment includes lithium, valproic acid, or an atypical antipsychotic; this is an acute manic episode. Because this patient has been experiencing a distinct period of elevated mood associated with grandiosity, decreased need for sleep, pressured speech, and increase in pleasure-seeking activities, his most likely diagnosis is BD I.

A 38-year-old woman presents to your office for an initial visit with a complaint of sleepiness during the day. She reports falling asleep easily and getting a full 8 hours of sleep every night. She is an otherwise healthy woman with a BMI of 19, and the only medication that she takes is a multivitamin. When questioned further, she reports a lack of energy and interest in many of her hobbies. What disorder(s) must be kept in mind?

Depression; there are multiple etiologies of "sleepiness" and the physician must re-evaluate the patient's medical history, medications, social situation, and other factors in order to make the proper diagnosis. Depressive disorders must be considered in the differential diagnosis of sleep disturbances. In this case, depression is likely. Primary hypersomnia does not necessarily coexist with mood symptoms and the patient does not present with a typical history seen in primary insomnia. She is less likely to have OSA given her female gender and normal weight. If depression exists, it may be primarily responsible for the sleep disturbance; thus initial treatment should target depression.

A 36-year-old woman with a history of hyperthyroidism, allergic rhinitis, and bipolar disorder (BD) presents with recent feelings of "sadness" and "blues." Her BD has been relatively well controlled on lithium. Over the course of the last month she began feeling "down" and initially ignored it because she thought it was due to her stressful job. She states that she hasn't been sleeping well lately and that she can hardly concentrate at work. When questioned further she admits to feelings of guilt. What is the next step in management of this patient?

Lithium, Symbax (combination of olanzapine and fluoxetine), quetiapine (Seroquel), and lamotrigine (Lamictal) can be used to treat depression in the context of BD. Given their potential to induce mania, antidepressants should be used with caution.

An 18-year-old man has recently started college. He does not leave his dorm room very much and seems disinterested by the activities around him. One day he buys a TV for everyone on his hall and makes plans to go around the world over winter break. His roommate notices that he is up most of the night working on "projects." What is the likely diagnosis?

BD I; this man's behavior—decreased need for sleep, excessive expenditures, increase in goal-directed activities—is characteristic of an acute manic episode.

A 35-year-old woman complains to her psychiatrist about feeling "moody" for the past few months. When asked to clarify, she describes a recent incident in which one of her friends did not invite her to a party, saying that she felt "crushed." She also states that she has no energy for anything because she feels as though she has been walking around with "heavy weights" strapped to her body. She appears very tired during the interview and later remarks that she has been sleeping "a lot more than usual." What is the likely diagnosis and subsequent treatment?

Atypical depression; atypical depression typically presents with hyperphagia, hypersomnia, leaden paralysis, reactive mood, and hypersensitivity to interpersonal rejection. Research suggests that MAOIs are effective for atypical depression.

A 23-year-old woman is seen in the ER and as the psychiatry consultant, you are told that her chief complaint is "only sleeping 2 hours per night." You assume that the woman will be exhausted and complaining of daytime sleepiness. To your surprise, she is typing away on her laptop and making many phone calls. After speaking with the patient, she confirms that she only sleeps a few hours every night, but that she doesn't feel the need to sleep any more than that. She also reports feeling very healthy overall, and she has even been refurnishing her entire apartment with new furniture and electronics until late at night for the past week. What is the likely diagnosis?

BD; the patient appears to be having a manic episode, which would suggest a diagnosis of BD. The patient should be questioned further. The important point here is that many psychiatric disorders will present with sleep-related complaints.

CHAPTER 3

Anxiety Disorders

INTRODUCTION

What is "anxiety"?

A subjective feeling of fear accompanied by physical symptoms

Is anxiety a normal human response?

Yes, and physicians must be careful when diagnosing patients with one of the anxiety disorders that the patient is not experiencing a normal, physiologic response to a possible threat.

What is the lifetime prevalence of anxiety disorders in men?

19%

What is the lifetime prevalence of anxiety disorders in women?

30%

What socioeconomic class is most predisposed to anxiety disorders?

Higher socioeconomic class

List some medical causes of anxiety.

- Hyperthyroidism
- Neurologic diseases including brain tumors and multiple sclerosis
- Vitamin B_{12} deficiency
- Anemia
- Pheochromocytoma
- Hypoglycemia
- Hypoxia

List some medications or substances that can induce anxiety.

- Caffeine
- Amphetamines
- Nicotine
- Cocaine
- Alcohol or sedative withdrawal
- Mercury or arsenic toxicity
- Antidepressants
- Organophosphate toxicity
- Penicillin or sulfonamides

PANIC DISORDER

What are the two major subtypes of panic disorder?

1. Panic disorder with agoraphobia
2. Panic disorder without agoraphobia

Is there a gender disparity in the diagnoses of panic disorder and agoraphobia?

Yes. They are more commonly diagnosed in women.

What is the typical age of onset?

Common in late teens to early thirties. Rarely, onset will be after 40.

! What do the majority of patients describe as the trigger for their first panic attack?

Nothing. Approximately 80% of patients cannot pinpoint a trigger for their first attack. A panic attack is typically the presenting feature of panic disorder.

What is a common childhood disorder that may predispose to the diagnosis of panic disorder as an adult?

A history of separation anxiety disorder is seen in 20%-50% of patients with an eventual diagnosis of panic disorder.

What are major comorbid psychiatric conditions seen in patients with panic disorder?

Major depression, substance abuse, social phobias, specific phobias, and obsessive-compulsive disorder (OCD)

! **How is a panic attack defined by *DSM-IV* (*Diagnostic and Statistical Manual of Mental Disorders, Fourth Edition*) criteria?**

A discrete period of intense fear or discomfort in which four of the following symptoms developed acutely and peaked in intensity within 10 minutes of onset:

- Palpitations or tachycardia
- Diaphoresis
- Sensation of shortness of breath
- Shaking or trembling
- Subjective feeling of choking
- Chest pain or discomfort
- Nausea or abdominal pain
- Lightheadedness or fainting
- Derealization (feelings of unreality) or depersonalization (being detached from oneself)
- Fear of losing control or going crazy
- Fear of dying
- Paresthesias
- Chills or warm sensations

What is the course of a typical panic attack?

They usually last between 20 and 30 minutes.

! **Which is more important in establishing the diagnosis of a panic attack: time to peak of symptoms or total length of symptoms?**

Time to peak

How often do panic attacks typically occur?

There is no typical frequency. They may occur many times per day or only a few times per year.

How is panic disorder diagnosed?

Panic disorder is characterized by multiple unexpected panic attacks **accompanied by anticipatory anxiety about having additional attacks.**

How may patients with panic disorder present to the emergency room?

With recurrent episodes of chest pain that mimic a myocardial infarction

What commonly used substances can exacerbate anxiety in patients both with and without panic disorder?

Caffeine and nicotine

What is panic disorder with agoraphobia?

Anxiety about being in public or a large space in which escape may be difficult or embarrassing, or in which help may not be readily available if one were to have an unexpected or situationally predisposed attack.

What is the differential diagnosis of panic disorder?

- *Medical:* myocardial infarction, angina, chronic obstructive pulmonary disease (COPD), congestive heart failure, pheochromocytoma; other cardiac, pulmonary, or endocrine disorders
- *Psychiatric:* depressive disorder, phobic disorders, OCD, posttraumatic stress disorder (PTSD)
- *Substance:* cocaine, nicotine, caffeine; alcohol or opiate withdrawal

How is panic disorder treated in the acute setting?

Symptomatically with anxiolytics, typically benzodiazepines such as lorazepam (Ativan)

What risk is associated with initial pharmacologic treatment of panic disorder?

Benzodiazepine dependence

! **How is panic disorder treated over the long-term?**

Tapered benzodiazepine dose (to avoid dependence) after initiation of long-term selective serotonin/norepinephrine reuptake inhibitor (SS/NRI) therapy

How is treatment of panic disorder with SS/NRIs different than treatment for depression?

Panic disorder is treated with **higher doses** of SS/NRIs.

What is the typical length of treatment with SS/NRIs for panic disorder?

These medications should be taken for 8-12 months as relapse of panic disorder is common.

What is an important side effect of SS/NRIs that should be explained to patients beginning to take them for panic disorder?

Patients may report anxiety, insomnia, and increased frequency of panic attacks upon initiation of SS/NRI therapy. This tends to resolve within the first week of treatment.

What is the best nonpharmacologic treatment for panic disorder?

Cognitive behavioral therapy (CBT) has been shown to be as effective as pharmacologic treatment.

SOCIAL ANXIETY DISORDER

What is a common activity during which social anxiety disorder becomes apparent?

Public speaking

! How is social anxiety disorder defined by *DSM-IV* criteria?

- Persistent and excessive fear of social or performance situations
- Exposure to the situation results in immediate anxiety
- The patient recognizes that the fear is excessive or unreasonable
- The avoidance or anticipation of the precipitating situation significantly interferes with the patient's routine
- The fear is not due to a general medical condition, substance induced, or due to another psychiatric disorder including panic attacks

How is social anxiety disorder treated?

High-dose SS/NRIs, CBT, and psychodynamic therapies have been shown to have some benefit.

! How would one distinguish between social anxiety disorder and avoidant personality disorder?

Social anxiety disorder involves an unreasonable **fear of embarrassment and humiliation** in social or performance situations, whereas avoidant personality disorder involves a **fear of rejection** in social situations.

SPECIFIC PHOBIA

What is a phobia?

An irrational fear that leads to avoidance

! How is specific phobia defined by DSM-I IV criteria?

- Persistent and excessive fear of a specific situation or thing.
- Exposure to the situation or thing results in immediate anxiety.
- The patient recognizes that the fear is excessive or unreasonable.
- The avoidance or anticipation of the precipitating situation or thing significantly interferes with the patient's routine.
- The fear is not due to a general medical condition, substance induced, or due to another psychiatric disorder including panic attacks.

What are some common specific phobias?
Fear of flying, fear of blood, fear of snakes, fear of heights

What is the gender disparity for diagnosed specific phobia?
Estimated to be twice as common in women as in men

How are specific phobias treated?
Achieve habituation or elimination of the fear response through systemic desensitization and supportive psychotherapy. Pharmacologic treatments have yet to show benefit.

What is systemic desensitization?
Gradually exposing patient to the feared situation while teaching relaxation techniques

How do some patients "self-treat"?
As with many other anxiety disorders, some patients will choose to drink alcohol to "lessen" their anxiety.

OBSESSIVE-COMPULSIVE DISORDER

What is OCD?
The presence of obsessions and/or compulsions that produce discomfort or impairment

When is the most common age of onset?
Early adulthood

Are women affected more than men?
No. Both genders are equally affected.

! **The occurrence of what other mental disorder in a first-degree relative predisposes a person to OCD?**
Tourette disorder

What is the etiology of OCD?
- *Genetic:* more common in patients who have first-degree relatives with OCD
- *Psychosocial:* the onset of OCD can be triggered by stressful events in up to 60% of patients

What is the physiologic basis of OCD?
Both abnormal regulation of serotonin and dysregulation in the basal ganglia-thalamo-cortical circuit have been implicated.

! **Define and differentiate obsessions and compulsions.**	*Obsessions:* Recurrent, repeated intrusive thoughts, ideas, or images. The patient attempts to suppress these thoughts and recognizes that they may be irrational. *Compulsions:* Repetitive conscious mental acts or ritual behaviors that a person feels driven to perform in response to an obsession. The patient recognizes that the behaviors are excessive and irrational. These rituals are generally disruptive and interfere with a person's daily activities. Performing the ritual temporarily relieves the anxiety.
How is OCD diagnosed?	Patients exhibit either obsessions **or** compulsions.
What percentage of OCD patients exhibit both obsessions and compulsions?	75%
Do patients with OCD have insight into their disorder?	Yes, patients usually recognize that they have irrational fears that they wish to get rid of.
What are some examples of compulsions?	Excessive hand-washing, checking locks, turning light switches on and off, counting things, skin picking (ie, dermatillomania), hair plucking (ie, trichotillomatia), nail biting (ie, onychophagia), and hoarding
How are the obsessions of OCD distinct from delusions?	The obsessions of OCD are experienced by patients as **ego-dystonic** (eg, a person with no history of violence has repeated thoughts of harming woman) and cause them significant distress.
! **How is OCD different from obsessive-compulsive personality disorder (OCPD)?**	OCPD is an Axis II diagnosis that pertains to patients who are overly obsessed with details and orderliness and generally do not perceive themselves to have a problem (poor insight).
What is the typical course of OCD?	Generally chronic with only about one-third of patients showing significant improvement

How is OCD treated?

Pharmacologic treatment combined with behavioral psychotherapy

What is the pharmacologic treatment of OCD?

SS/NRIs at **higher doses** than those used for the treatment of depression and other disorders. Tricyclic antidepressants (TCAs), specifically clomipramine (Anafranil), have also shown some efficacy.

How is behavioral therapy conducted?

Exposure to ritual-eliciting situations and prevention of the resulting compulsions

What surgical procedure has been used in the treatment of intractable OCD?

Anterior cingulotomy

POSTTRAUMATIC STRESS DISORDER

What is PTSD?

The response to a traumatic or stressful life event in which the patient reexperiences the event, avoids similar situations or reminders, and may experience hyperarousal or emotional blunting

! **Is the response immediate or delayed (in relation to the inciting event)?**

It can be either immediate or delayed (ie, up to years after the initial traumatic event).

What are examples of people who may have PTSD?

War veterans, rape victims, mugging victims

! **What are the *DSM-IV* criteria for PTSD?**

- The person experiences an event that involved death, serious threat to life, or bodily harm that was experienced with intense fear, horror, or hopelessness.
- The traumatic event is persistently reexperienced in dreams or flashbacks.
- There is repeated avoidance of the stimuli associated with the trauma.
- Persistent symptoms of increased arousal including hypervigilance, insomnia, irritability, and so on.
- Symptoms persist for at least 1 month and cause distress or impairment in functioning.

What are common comorbid conditions in patients with PTSD?

Substance abuse and depression

How is PTSD generally treated?

A combination of pharmacologic and behavioral therapy

What drugs are used in the treatment of PTSD?

SS/NRIs, MAOIs (monoamine oxidase inhibitors), TCAs, benzodiazepines, and mood stabilizers

What medications, if used in the acute period following exposure to trauma, have been found to reduce the severity of PTSD symptoms over the long-term?

Beta-blockers

What are some behavioral therapies that have shown efficacy?

Exposure therapy, group therapy, CBT, eye movement desensitization and reprocessing (EMDR), and psychodynamic therapy

What is EMDR?

It involves the patient recalling and visualizing the traumatic experience while making repeated eye movements. EMDR has been found to be equally effective to pharmacotherapy and exposure therapy in multiple RCTs and meta-analyses.

Is "debriefing" found to be effective in reducing the development of PTSD?

No. Multiple studies have found that debriefing, which involves encouraging the recollection of the traumatic event for the sake of emotional processing, may increase the risk of PTSD and depression.

What medication has been found to be effective in reducing the nightmares associated with PTSD?

Prazosin

ACUTE STRESS DISORDER

What is acute stress disorder?

A disorder similar to PTSD where the patient has exhibited symptoms for only a short duration

How would acute stress disorder be diagnosed?
Symptoms are identical to those in PTSD but the inciting event must have occurred less than 1 month ago, and symptoms must have been present for less than 1 month. As in PTSD, the response to the traumatic event must cause impairment in functioning.

What happens if the symptoms of acute stress disorder persist for more than 1 month?
The diagnosis of PTSD is usually made.

How is acute stress disorder treated?
Same as for PTSD. Also brief supportive psychotherapy can be used.

GENERALIZED ANXIETY DISORDER

What is generalized anxiety disorder (GAD)?
GAD is characterized by excessive and uncontrollable worry about life circumstances accompanied by hyperarousal.

What percentage of patients with GAD are diagnosed with another anxiety disorder during their lifetime?
80%

What gender, age, ethnicity, and socioeconomic group are most predisposed to GAD?
Young to middle aged, nonwhite females in lower socioeconomic classes

How much more commonly is GAD observed in women as compared to men?
Approximately twice as common in women

! What are the diagnostic features of GAD according to the *DSM-IV*?

- Excessive worry or anxiety about several life events or activities for at least 6 months
- Difficulty controlling the worry
- At least three of the following symptoms are present when anxious:
  - Muscle tension
  - Easy fatigability
  - Restlessness
  - Irritability
  - Difficulty falling or staying asleep
  - Difficulty concentrating
- The worry must be out of proportion to the likelihood or impact of feared events
- Symptoms are not attributable to other medical or psychiatric conditions

! Upon interviewing patients with suspected GAD, what do they generally report regarding their life?

Many patients report being anxious for as long as they can remember.

What is the most effective therapeutic approach to GAD?

A combination of pharmacologic therapy with psychotherapy (especially CBT)

What medications are shown to be beneficial?

Buspirone (BuSpar, a nonbenzodiazepine anxiolytic), benzodiazepines, and **high-dose** SS/NRIs

What is the best nonpharmalogic treatment for GAD?

Cognitive behavioral therapy (CBT) has been shown to be as effective as pharmacotherapy for GAD.

! If a history of alcohol abuse exists, what medications should be avoided?

Benzodiazepines

ADJUSTMENT DISORDERS

Are adjustment disorders considered anxiety disorders?

Technically they are not. Adjustment disorders describe maladaptive responses to stressful life events.

! **What are the diagnostic features of adjustment disorders according to the *DSM-IV*?**

- The development of emotional or behavioral symptoms within 3 months of a life stressor and the cessation of these symptoms within 6 months after the stressor has passed.
- The symptoms produce distress out of proportion to the stressor and cause social impairment.

How is the course of an adjustment disorder useful in differentiating it from other anxiety and mood disorders?

Symptoms of adjustment disorder resolve **within 6 months after termination of the stressor(s)**. If symptoms persist, think of an anxiety disorder, PTSD, or mood disorder.

What are the different subtypes of adjustment disorders and how are they classified?

Classification is based on the predominant symptom: depressed mood, aggressive conduct, anxiety, and so on.

What is the gender predominance?

Females are affected twice as often as males, but it should be noted that the overall prevalence of adjustment disorders in the population is quite low.

How are adjustment disorders treated?

Supportive psychotherapy. Pharmacotherapy for the associated symptoms is also effective.

CLINICAL VIGNETTES

A 34-year-old African American mother of four comes into your office complaining of back pain, difficulty sleeping, and irritability. When you ask what has been happening in her life lately, she responds with a list of concerns such as getting the kids to school on time, making sure the house is clean, and getting the freshest foods for her kids. She claims that she has been worrying about these things for years and says that her mother always called her a "worry-wart." What is the likely diagnosis?

Generalized anxiety disorder (GAD); the patient describes excessive worry about everyday events and also reports constitutional symptoms such as muscle pain and irritability. Most importantly, the patient describes herself as a "worrier" and reports that these worries and symptoms have been long standing. All of these characteristics are consistent with GAD.

What is the best treatment plan for the patient in the previous vignette?

The most effective way to treat GAD is psychotherapy in combination with medications (either high-dose SS/NRIs, buspirone [Buspar], or a benzodiazepine).

A 51-year-old man enters the ER complaining of chest pain, palpitations, sweating, and dizziness. He says that he feels like he is "dying." What is at the top of your differential diagnosis?

A myocardial infarction *must* be ruled out; although this man could be having a panic attack, a myocardial infarction presents similarly and must be worked up before the appropriate panic disorder workup.

A 37-year-old businessman is leaving work one afternoon when he suddenly feels his heart beating quickly "through his chest," breaks into a cold sweat, and feels a huge lump in his throat. He thinks he is having a heart attack and might be dying. After loosening his tie and sitting down, he feels better after 20 minutes. What is the likely diagnosis, and what is the proper treatment if it were to happen again?

Panic attack; as the symptoms became apparent in a very acute fashion and peaked quickly, panic attack is the most likely diagnosis. If it occurred again, he could take a benzodiazepine such as lorazepam (Ativan) or klonazepam (Klonopin) for short-term treatment.

A 31-year-old consultant is about to make a presentation to a prospective client. Outside of the conference room he begins to hyperventilate and perspire. He sits on the ground and cannot bring himself to enter the room. What is the likely diagnosis and the best treatment course?

Social phobia manifested by public speaking; SS/NRIs are first-line treatment. Some patients with this type of performance anxiety have also been treated acutely with betablockers (eg, propranolol) or benzodiazepines.

A 24-year-old lieutenant who recently returned from combat in Iraq comes into your office complaining of feeling scared every time he drives. He said that this fear began 3 or 4 days ago, and he has been back from the war for only 3 weeks. When he drives, he describes "heightened senses" as well as flashbacks to driving in Iraq and seeing roadside landmines explode. What is the diagnosis?

The diagnosis of posttraumatic stress disorder (PTSD) versus acute stress disorder (ASD) cannot be precisely determined at this point; given that the symptoms have lasted only a few days, a diagnosis of PTSD cannot be firmly established as it requires persistent symptoms for more than 4 weeks. The symptomatology of PTSD and ASD are the same, but ASD is likely the correct diagnosis in this case. If his symptoms lasted another 2 weeks, then PTSD would be the correct diagnosis.

A 19-year-old man takes 2 hours to clean and dress himself in the morning. When he is ready to leave the house, he stands in the doorway and must turn the light switch off, then on again, then off, and so on. He does this exactly 200 times before he can leave the house. He claims that if he does not turn the light on and off 200 times, his apartment will catch on fire while he is gone. What is the diagnosis? How would you describe its components?

Obsessive-compulsive disorder; the obsession is a recurrent and intrusive thought of the man's apartment catching on fire, and the compulsion is his ritualized light-switching in hopes that it will "combat" the obsession. This clearly leads to significant disruption of the man's daily activities. Appropriate treatment includes pharmacologic therapy with SS/NRIs (at higher does than those used for depression) or clomipramine (Anafranil) in combination with cognitive behavioral therapy.

A 27-year-old law student comes to her primary care physician complaining of a rapid heart beat, abdominal pain, diarrhea, and lightheadedness almost every morning over the past week. These symptoms tend to lessen in severity during the course of the day, but are very troublesome to her. She recognizes that exams are "stressing her out," but she says that tests never worried her before. Before making the diagnosis of panic attacks or panic disorder, what habits should the physician inquire about?

Caffeine intake and cigarette smoking (in addition to other drug use); these substances can contribute significantly to anxiety and its systemic symptoms. Their use should be limited if panic disorder is a suspected diagnosis.

CHAPTER 4

Psychotic Disorders

INTRODUCTION

What is psychosis?

Abnormal condition of the mind involving delusions, perceptual disturbances, and/or disordered thinking and behavior

What types of thought disorders exist?

- Thought content—reflect patients' beliefs, ideas, and interpretations
- Thought process—reflect manner in which patients link ideas and words together

! **What are examples of disorders of thought content?**

- Delusions—fixed, false beliefs that are not shared by the person's culture and cannot be changed by reasoning
- Suicidal and homicidal thoughts
- Phobias—persistent, irrational fears
- Obsessions—repetitive, intrusive thoughts
- Compulsions—repetitive behaviors
- Poverty of thought versus overabundance—too few versus too many ideas expressed

What are examples of disorders of thought process?

- Loose associations—no logical relationship between thoughts
- Flight of ideas—a stream of very tangential thoughts
- Tangentiality—lack of goal-directed associations between ideas; point of conversation never reached
- Circumstantiality—point of conversation is reached after roundabout path
- Thought blocking—abrupt termination of communication before the idea is finished
- Clang associations—word associations due to sounds instead of actual meaning (You are tall. I hope I don't fall. Let's go to the mall.)
- Neologisms—fabricated words
- Word salad—unintelligible collection of words

What are the types of delusions?

- Paranoid—false belief that one is being targeted unfairly ("The government is recording my conversations.")
- Ideas of reference—false belief that events have special personal significance ("The President of the United States speaks to me through the TV.")
- Thought broadcasting—false belief that one's thoughts are transmitted to everyone
- Delusions of grandeur—false belief that the individual is much greater and more powerful and influential than he or she really is ("I am the son of God.")
- Delusions of guilt—false belief that one is guilty or responsible for something ("I am responsible for the tsunami.")
- Somatic delusions—false belief that a part of one's body has been injured or altered in some manner ("My body is rotting away.")
- Erotomanic delusions—false belief that one is the love interest of someone of higher status, for example, a celebrity

! What are examples of perceptual disturbances?

- Hallucinations—sensory experiences that arise in the absence of a direct external stimulus (visual, auditory, tactile, gustatory, olfactory)
- Illusions—misinterpretation of existing sensory stimuli (eg, an inanimate object appears to move)

SCHIZOPHRENIA

Epidemiology and Etiology

What is the lifetime prevalence of schizophrenia?

1%

Are there any gender disparities in the incidence of schizophrenia?

No

! What is the typical age of onset?

~20 years for men, ~30 years for women

Is there a genetic predisposition for schizophrenia?

Yes. 50% concordance among monozygotic twins, 10% risk if one first-degree relative is affected.

! What socioeconomic groups are most at risk for schizophrenia?

Lower socioeconomic groups. Some authors argue that this association is due to "downward drift," or that schizophrenia causes one to have a downward shift in social class.

What neurotransmitter abnormalities are implicated in schizophrenia?

Elevated dopamine, elevated serotonin, and decreased *N*-methyl-D-aspartic acid; glutamate (NMD A) receptor function

What evidence supports the dopamine hypothesis of schizophrenia?

Increased dopaminergic activity from drugs such as amphetamines and levodopa causes psychosis. Postsynaptic dopamine blockade improves psychotic symptoms.

What dopamine pathways are thought to be affected in schizophrenia?

Prefrontal (negative symptoms) and mesolimbic (positive symptoms) pathways

What structural imaging findings are characteristic of schizophrenia?

Ventricular enlargement, reduced temporal lobe volume, and diffuse cortical atrophy

! **What percent of schizophrenic patients commit suicide?**

~10%

Diagnosis

! **What are the *DSM-IV* (*Diagnostic and Statistical Manual of Mental Disorders, Fourth Edition*) criteria for diagnosing schizophrenia?**

- Two or more of the following must be present for at least 1 month:
  - Delusions
  - Hallucinations
  - Disorganized speech
  - Grossly disorganized or catatonic behavior
  - Negative symptoms
- Must cause significant social or occupational functional deterioration
- Duration of illness for at least 6 months (including prodromal or residual symptoms in which above criteria may not be met)
- Symptoms not due to medical, neurologic, or substance-induced disorder

What are the positive symptoms of schizophrenia?

Hallucinations, delusions, bizarre behavior, and thought disorder

! **What are the negative symptoms of schizophrenia?**

5 **A**'s

Anhedonia

Affect (flat)

Alogia (poverty of speech)

Avolition (apathy)

Attention (poor)

What is the differential diagnosis of schizophrenia?

Brief psychotic disorder, psychotic disorder due to general medical conditions, substance-induced psychotic disorders, **mood disorders with psychotic features,** schizoaffective disorders, schizophreniform disorder, delusional disorder, autism, and obsessive-compulsive disorder

What recreational drugs can cause symptoms that mimic acute schizophrenia?

Cocaine, methamphetamine, phencyclidine (PCP), and ketamine

What prescription drugs can cause psychotic symptoms?

Fluoroquinolones, dextromethorphan, antihistamines, **steroids**, anticholinergic drugs, **L-dopa**

What are the three phases of schizophrenia?

1. *Prodromal*—decline in functioning that precedes first psychotic episode
2. *Psychotic*—positive symptoms
3. *Residual*—exists between psychotic episodes and marked by negative symptoms, although hallucinations may persist

What are the subtypes of schizophrenia?

- *Disorganized*—disorganized speech/behavior, flat/inappropriate affect. Low functioning, worse prognosis than other subtypes
- *Catatonic*—motor immobility/excessive purposeless motor activity, extreme mutism, echolalia (repeats words), echopraxia (repeats movements); rare
- *Paranoid*—delusions/hallucinations present, but no predominance of disorganized or catatonic behavior, and cognitive function typically preserved. High functioning, better prognosis than other subtypes
- *Undifferentiated*—characteristics of more than one subtype or none of the subtypes
- *Residual*—prominent negative symptoms with minimal positive symptoms

! **What is the typical course of schizophrenia?**

Prominent deterioration in first 5-10 years of illness, often followed by a long plateau. Schizophrenia is usually chronic and debilitating. Forty to fifty percent of patients remain significantly impaired, while 20%-30% function fairly well with medication.

! **What features of the disease are associated with a better prognosis?**

Later onset, good social support, positive symptoms, mood symptoms, acute onset, female sex, few relapses, and good premorbid functioning

! **What features of the disease are associated with a worse prognosis?**	Early onset, poor social support, negative symptoms, family history, gradual onset, male sex, many relapses, ventricular enlargement, and poor premorbid functioning
What are some of the typical findings in schizophrenic patients on examination?	Disheveled appearance, flattened affect, disorganized thought process, intact memory and orientation, auditory hallucinations, paranoid delusions, ideas of reference, concrete understanding of similarities/proverbs, and lack of insight into their disease

Treatment (*see Chapter 14 for more detailed information on treatment*)

What classes of medications are used to treat schizophrenia?	Typical and atypical antipsychotics
List some typical antipsychotics.	Chlorpromazine (Thorazine), thioridazine (Mellaril), trifluoperazine (Stelazine), haloperidol (Haldol)
List some atypical antipsychotics.	Risperidone (Risperdal), clozapine (Clozaril), olanzapine (Zyprexa), quetiapine (Seroquel), aripiprazole (Abilify), ziprasidone (Geodon)
! **How do typical and atypical antipsychotics differ in their side effect profile?**	• Typical antipsychotics are thought to have a greater association with movement disorders (eg, EPS and tardive dyskinesia). • Atypical antipsychotics are thought to have a greater association with metabolic side effects (eg, weight gain, high cholesterol, insulin resistance).
! **Which antipsychotics are most effective in treating psychosis?**	According to the CATIE trial, all typical and atypical antipsychotics are equally effective, with the exception of clozapine (Clozaril), which is more effective in treatment-refractory schizophrenia.
What adjunct treatments can be useful for patients with schizophrenia?	Cognitive behavioral therapy helps patients find alternative ways of understanding and managing the hallucinations and delusions of psychosis. Family and group therapy are also useful.

What are the indications for electroconvulsive therapy (ECT) in schizophrenia?	Catatonia, prominent mood symptoms, medication-refractory symptoms, and acute-severe psychosis

SCHIZOPHRENIFORM DISORDER

! **What are the criteria for diagnosing schizophreniform disorder?**	Same as schizophrenia, **but symptoms have lasted for only 1-6 months**
! **What is the diagnosis when symptoms last for more than 6 months?**	Schizophrenia
! **What is the diagnosis when symptoms last for less than 1 month?**	Brief psychotic disorder
What is the typical course of schizophreniform disorder?	One-third of patients recover completely; two-thirds progress to schizoaffective disorder or schizophrenia
What are the prognostic factors for schizophreniform disorder?	Same as schizophrenia
What treatment options are available for a person with schizophreniform disorder?	Hospitalization, 3- to 6-month course of antipsychotics, and supportive psychotherapy

SCHIZOAFFECTIVE DISORDER

! **What are the *DSM-IV* criteria for diagnosing schizoaffective disorder?**	• Both a mood episode and the psychotic features of schizophrenia are present simultaneously during any uninterrupted period of mental illness. • Delusions or hallucinations are present for 2 weeks in the absence of mood disorder symptoms during same uninterrupted period. • Mood symptoms are present for substantial portion of psychotic illness.
! **What is the minimum duration of time for diagnosing schizoaffective disorder?**	1 month

What are the two types of schizoaffective disorder?

Bipolar and depressive types, depending on which type of mood episode predominates

What is the prognosis of schizoaffective disorder?

Better than schizophrenia but worse than mood disorders

What are the treatment options for schizoaffective disorder?

- Antipsychotics for short-term control of psychosis; mood stabilizers, antidepressants, or ECT as needed for mania or depression
- Hospitalization and supportive psychotherapy

! **How does one distinguish between schizoaffective disorder and mood disorder with psychotic features?**

In schizoaffective disorder, psychotic symptoms predominate (Think: "**schizo**affective," ie, schizophrenic symptoms before affective symptoms) and must be present for at least two weeks without the presence of mood symptoms. In a mood disorder with psychotic features, mood symptoms (ie, mania or depression) predominate.

BRIEF PSYCHOTIC DISORDER

! **What are the criteria for diagnosing brief psychotic disorder?**

Same as defined for schizophrenia, but **duration of symptoms is 1 day to 1 month.**

What is the typical course of brief psychotic disorder?

50%-80% recover; remainder may eventually be diagnosed with schizophrenia or mood disorder

What is the treatment for brief psychotic disorder?

Brief hospitalization, a course of antipsychotics or benzodiazepines, and supportive psychotherapy

What is the prognosis of brief psychotic disorder as compared to other psychiatric disorders?

From best to worst prognosis: mood disorder > brief psychotic disorder > schizoaffective disorder > schizophreniform disorder > schizophrenia

! Use duration of illness to distinguish between brief psychotic disorder, schizophreniform disorder, and schizophrenia.

<1 month symptoms	Brief psychotic disorder
1-6 months symptoms	Schizophreniform disorder
>6 months symptoms	Schizophrenia

DELUSIONAL DISORDER

! What are the *DSM-IV* criteria for diagnosing delusional disorder?

- **Nonbizarre**, fixed delusions for at least 1 month
- Does not meet criteria for schizophrenia
- Auditory or visual hallucinations are not prominent
- Daily functioning is not significantly impaired

What are the subtypes of delusional disorder?

- Erotomanic type: romantic preoccupation with a stranger
- Grandiose type: inflated self-worth
- Somatic type: physical delusions
- Persecutory type: delusions of being persecuted
- Jealous type: delusions of infidelity
- Mixed type: more than one of the above

What is the typical course of delusional disorder?

50% recovery, 20% decreased symptoms, and 30% no change

What is the treatment for delusional disorder?

Psychotherapy and antipsychotic medications

! What features differentiate schizophrenia from delusional disorder?

- Delusions in delusional disorder are nonbizarre and do not occur in the presence of other psychotic symptoms.
- In delusional disorder, daily functioning is not impaired.

What distinguishes bizarre from nonbizarre delusions?

- *Nonbizarre delusions*—beliefs that might occur in real life but are not currently true (eg, having an unfaithful spouse)
- *Bizarre delusions*—beliefs that have no basis in reality (eg, believing that aliens are controlling the world)

SHARED PSYCHOTIC DISORDER (or "Folie á deux")

What are the *DSM-IV* criteria for diagnosing shared psychotic disorder (or "folie á deux")?

A patient develops the same delusional symptoms as someone he or she is in a close relationship with. This typically occurs among family members.

What is the prognosis for shared psychotic disorder?

20%-40% will recover upon separation from the inducing person.

What is the treatment of shared psychotic disorder?

- Separate the patient from the person who is the source of the shared delusions.
- Psychotherapy.
- Prescribe antipsychotic medications if symptoms have not improved 1-2 weeks after separation.

OTHER PSYCHOTIC DISORDERS AND SYNDROMES

What are the *DSM-IV* criteria for diagnosing substance-induced psychotic disorder?

Psychotic symptoms developed during/within a month of substance intoxication or withdrawal; or medication use is etiologically related to the symptoms.

What are the *DSM-IV* criteria for diagnosing psychotic disorder not otherwise specified (NOS)?

Psychotic symptoms that do not meet full criteria for a specific disorder, or psychotic symptoms without enough information to make a specific diagnosis

What are the criteria for diagnosing postpartum psychosis?

Psychosis in close temporal association with childbirth

! What symptoms characterize postpartum psychosis?

Depression, delusions, thoughts by the mother of harming the infant or herself, cognitive deficits, and occasional hallucinations. **This is a psychiatric emergency, usually requiring hospitalization of the mother to prevent harm to herself or the infant.**

What is Capgras syndrome?

The belief that people have been replaced by imposters

What is Cotard syndrome?

Nihilistic delusion in which people believe that they are dead or do not exist

What is Fregoli syndrome?

The belief that different people are in fact a single person who changes appearance or is in disguise

What is koro?

Belief that one's external genitals (ie, penis or nipples) are retracting or shrinking and will eventually disappear. It is a culture-bound syndrome mostly found in China and Southeast Asia.

CLINICAL VIGNETTES

A 22-year-old woman was diagnosed with schizophrenia after one episode of psychosis (auditory hallucinations and paranoid delusions) that lasted 9 months. She was immediately started on risperidone and since then has been symptom free for 18 months. What treatment change(s), if any, should be made?

Since the patient had only one episode of psychosis and has been symptom free for over 1 year, and given the adverse effects of antipsychotic medications (such as metabolic syndrome and movement disorders), her physician should minimize and, if possible, discontinue the medication. This should be done gradually, with frequent visits to her psychiatrist, so as to reduce the risk of relapse.

A 20-year-old man is brought to the emergency department (ED) after refusing to eat any food for almost a week. He tearfully states that the government has been poisoning all the food in his family's household. He admits to having attempted suicide recently, and claims that he would be "better off dead." He has been expressing these fears regarding the government for the last 6 months. What is the likely diagnosis?

Schizoaffective disorder, depressive type; this disorder involves at least 1 month of simultaneous mood disorder and psychotic symptoms, and at least one 2-week period where the patient experiences psychotic symptoms in the absence of mood symptoms.

A 35-year-old woman has been diagnosed with schizophrenia for 10 years. She has complained of persistent hallucinations, such as constantly hearing voices that tell her to kill herself. She states that at this point, she has "gotten used to it." She believes that her family is being targeted by the Taliban, and she worries whether she will "make it through the year alive." She does not display disorganized thought or behavior. She has managed to hold a low-paying job over the years. What subtype of schizophrenia does this woman suffer from? What prognosis is this subtype associated with?

Schizophrenia, paranoid subtype. Better prognosis than other subtypes; this subtype is associated with delusions and hallucinations, but has no predominance of disorganized or catatonic behavior. Patients with this subtype tend to be higher functioning. Patients with the disorganized subtype of schizophrenia tend to be lower functioning and have a worse prognosis.

A patient with schizophrenia presents to the ED with persistent hyponatremia and low urine specific gravity. He complains of frequent urination. What is the likely diagnosis and subsequent management?

Psychogenic polydipsia; restrict water intake; self-induced water intoxication should always be considered in the differential diagnosis of confusional states and seizures in schizophrenia patients; as many as 20% of schizophrenic patients drink water excessively. Medications such as lithium and carbamazepine, which cause water retention, can aggravate these symptoms.

A 21-year-old man is brought to the ED after exhibiting "erratic" behavior. For the last 4 months, he has become increasingly suspicious of the people around him, particularly his parents. He has barricaded himself in his bedroom, and his parents have overheard him shouting at "no one in particular." In his answers to the attending physicians he is noted to jump from topic to topic randomly. His speech is frequently incoherent, and at other times, he complains of hearing voices that instruct him to harm his parents. What is the diagnosis?

Schizophreniform disorder; this patient has had the symptoms of schizophrenia for between 1 and 6 months.

A 27-year-old man recently diagnosed with schizophrenia presents for his initial evaluation. He is accompanied by his parents. They state that he has been acting strangely for months, even years. They describe him as becoming progressively more withdrawn. They allege that he has become more and more "apathetic"; for example, he recently quit his job and no longer attends to his basic hygienic needs. On questioning, he appears indifferent; he describes the recent death of a friend in a monotone. He exhibits flight of ideas and ideas of reference. His parents state that even when he was much younger, he did not perform well in school and had few friends. Despite this, they are eager to help their son with his troubles. According to the details of this man's presentation, what sort of prognosis can be expected?

Poor prognosis; many aspects of the man's presentation point toward a poor prognosis: male sex, insidious onset of schizophrenia, poor premorbid functioning, and prominent negative symptoms. The man's strong social support (in the form of his parents) is associated with a good prognosis. Other features that would be associated with a good prognosis are later onset, positive symptoms, mood symptoms, acute onset, female sex, few relapses, and good premorbid functioning.

A 19-year-old woman has been exhibiting strange behavior over the last 2 weeks. Her father has overheard her talking to herself while no one is in the room. She also claims to be having "visions" involving "tiny men and women patrolling her bedroom." Her father believes that she may be very stressed out, as she is studying hard for her final exams. Her symptoms continue until she finishes her exams, after which her strange behavior ceases completely. She reports no further symptoms. What is the diagnosis?

Brief psychotic disorder; this person has had psychotic symptoms for less than 1 month followed by full spontaneous remission. Brief psychotic disorder is characterized by the sudden appearance of psychotic symptoms, usually following a severe stressor (in this woman's case, her final exams).

A 50-year-old physician has been complaining to his colleagues that his wife is "cheating" on him. Despite no evidence to support this, and despite his wife's repeated assurances that she has been faithful, he states "I know she's been fooling around." During this time, the physician has not neglected his professional duties. What is the likely diagnosis?

Delusional disorder; this disorder is typified by "nonbizarre" delusions and the absence of other psychotic symptoms. Daily functioning is not significantly impaired.

A 29-year-old mother of two young children is taken to the hospital after her husband reports hearing her yelling while she is alone in the backyard. He tells the physician that the patient has been very sad lately, displayed a lack of energy, has had difficulty sleeping, and has lost weight but that these symptoms apparently abated over 1 month ago. He has heard her talk to herself throughout the past months, but he hoped that it "was nothing big." What is the likely diagnosis?

Schizoaffective disorder; this diagnosis is likely because the psychotic symptoms in this case, auditory hallucinations, have persisted for more than 2 weeks since her mood disorder seemingly resolved.

What would the differential diagnosis be if the patient above were to present with depressive symptoms concurrent with the psychotic features?

Depression with psychotic features or schizoaffective disorder; if the psychotic and depressive symptoms were concurrent, one would not be able to distinguish between these two diagnoses at that point.

A 25-year-old woman has been diagnosed with schizophrenia for the past 5 years. She has tried various antipsychotic medications with no success; she still experiences psychotic symptoms on a daily basis. What medication might be appropriate for her? What additional measures must be taken with this drug?

Clozapine (Clozaril) is the best choice for treatment of refractory schizophrenia. Patients on clozapine (Clozaril) must have regular CBCs to check for agranulocytosis, which occurs in 1%-2% of all patients on this medication. Other side effects seen in particular with clozapine (Clozaril) are decreased seizure threshold (risk increases at >600 mg daily), tachycardia, myocarditis, sialorrhea (drooling), and transient hyperthermia.

You have been treating a 35-year-old man for schizophrenia with Risperdal 8 mg at bedtime for several months. During his most recent appointment, you notice that he has developed some strange movements in his face that look like "lip smacking." What is happening and how can it be treated?

Tardive dyskinesia (TD), which consists of darting or writhing movements of the face, tongue, and head. This is a movement side effect of antipsychotics that develops over the course of months of treatment. The only treatment choices are to switch to another agent (clozapine [Clozaril] is the least likely to cause TD) or stop the offending agent.

A 25-year-old obese male presents to your office for treatment for schizophrenia. He tells you that he would like to try one of "those newer antipsychotic medications. I've heard they are better." How would you respond?

You should tell him that most research shows that all antipsychotic medications are equally effective for treating schizophrenia except for clozapine (Clozaril), which is more effective for "treatment refractory" schizophrenia. You could inform him that side effects are often a good way to choose between these medications. Although many patients (and clinicians, for that matter) are excited to use newer ("atypical") antipsychotics, most of these medications (save aripiprazole [Abilify] and, to a lesser extent, ziprasidone [Geodon]) are known to cause metabolic syndrome (hyperlipidemia, impaired glucose metabolism, and weight gain). Since this patient is already obese, most atypicals may not be a good choice. Typical antipsychotics are as effective and many (such as haloperidol [Haldol]) have less propensity for weight gain, making them another option.

CHAPTER 5

Personality Disorders

OVERVIEW

What is meant by personality?

A person's set of stable, predictable emotional and behavioral traits

What is meant by personality disorder?

Long-term, stable pattern of maladaptive and **inflexible** personality traits that leads to **impairment or distress**.

What is the prevalence of personality disorders?

10%-20% of the general population. It is higher in psychiatric patients (30%-50%).

What is the typical age of onset of personality disorders?

DSM-IV (*Diagnostic and Statistical Manual of Mental Disorders, Fourth Edition*) definition requires an onset no later than early adulthood. However, some individuals' personality disorders may not come to clinical attention until later in life.

! **What are the *DSM-IV* diagnostic criteria for personality disorders?**

- Pattern of behavior/inner experience that deviates from the person's culture and is manifested in two or more of the following ways:
  - Cognition
  - Affect
  - Personal relations
  - Impulse control
- Pattern:
  - Is pervasive and inflexible in a broad range of situations
  - Is stable and has an onset no later than adolescence or early adulthood
  - Is not accounted for by another mental/medical illness or by use of a substance

! What are some ways in which the assessment of patients with personality disorders is unique?

- It is often necessary **to conduct more than one interview with patients and to space these over time**, since a personality disorder is defined as a stable, inflexible way of interacting with others.
- Assessment can also be complicated by the fact that the characteristics defining a personality disorder may not be considered problematic by the individual (ie, the traits are often **ego-syntonic**).
- Be sure to rule out Axis I disorders first.

What are some clues to the diagnosis of personality disorder?

- Impaired interpersonal relations.
- Externalization of blame, that is, "It's not my fault."
- Failure to learn from past mistakes.
- Physician countertransference: conscious or unconscious emotional response of the therapist to the individual, including feelings of irritation, frustration, anger, or being manipulated.

! What are the three clusters of personality disorders?

3 **W**s

Cluster A (**"Weird"**): paranoid, schizoid, and schizotypal

- Eccentric, peculiar, or withdrawn
- Familial association with psychotic disorders

Cluster B (**"Wild"**): antisocial, borderline, histrionic, and narcissistic

- Emotional, dramatic, or erratic
- Familial association with mood disorders

Cluster C (**"Worried"**): avoidant, dependent, and obsessive-compulsive

- Anxious or fearful
- Familial association with anxiety disorders

What "Axis" are personality disorders grouped under in the DSM?

Axis II

How are personality disorders generally treated?

Personality disorders can be difficult to treat, as few patients are aware that they need help and these disorders tend to be chronic. **Group and individual psychotherapy are the mainstays of treatment**. Pharmacologic treatment is used mostly for comorbid conditions (eg, depression and anxiety).

CLUSTER A ("WEIRD")

Paranoid Personality Disorder

What other psychiatric diseases are more commonly seen among relatives of individuals with PPD?

Schizophrenia and delusional disorder

What are the *DSM-IV* diagnostic criteria for PPD?

General distrust of others, beginning by early adulthood and present in a variety of contexts. At least four of the following must also be present:

- Suspicion (without evidence) that others are exploiting or deceiving him or her
- Preoccupation with doubts of loyalty or trustworthiness of acquaintances
- Reluctance to confide in others
- Interpretation of benign remarks as threatening or demeaning
- Persistence of grudges
- Perception of attacks on his or her character that are not apparent to others; quick to counterattack
- Recurrence of suspicions regarding fidelity of spouse or lover

What is the differential diagnosis of PPD?

Psychotic disorders with persecutory delusions (especially paranoid schizophrenia), delusional disorder, personality changes due to general medical conditions, substance-induced personality changes, and other personality disorders

! **What is the difference between paranoid schizophrenia and PPD?**

People with PPD do not have fixed delusions and are not frankly psychotic, although they may have transient psychosis under stressful situations.

What is the typical course of PPD?

PPD tends to have a chronic course; symptoms may intensify later in life with social/sensory isolation. Some patients may eventually be diagnosed with schizophrenia or delusional disorder.

How is PPD treated?

Psychotherapy is the mainstay of treatment. Antipsychotic or antianxiety medications can be useful for transient psychosis.

Schizoid Personality Disorder

What is the prevalence of schizoid PD?

7%

What are the *DSM-IV* diagnostic criteria for schizoid PD?

A pattern of **voluntary social withdrawal** and restricted range of emotional expression, beginning by early adulthood and present in a variety of contexts. Four or more of the following must also be present:

- Neither enjoying nor desiring close relationships (including family)
- Generally choosing solitary activities
- Little (if any) interest in sexual activity with another person
- Taking pleasure in few activities (if any)
- Few close friends or confidants (if any)
- Indifference to praise or criticism
- Emotional coldness, detachment, or flattened affect

What is the differential diagnosis of schizoid PD?

Residual symptoms in schizophrenia, autistic disorder, Asperger disorder, and other personality disorders

How is schizoid PD treated?

Psychotherapy is the treatment of choice. Short-term antipsychotic or antidepressant medications can be used for transient psychosis or comorbid depression.

Schizotypal Personality Disorder

What psychiatric diseases are more commonly seen among relatives of individuals with schizotypal PD?

Schizotypal PD and schizophrenia

What are the *DSM-IV* diagnostic criteria for schizotypal PD?

A pattern of social deficits marked by **eccentric behavior**, cognitive or perceptual distortions, and discomfort with close relationships, beginning by early adulthood and present in a variety of contexts. Five or more of the following must be present:
- Ideas of reference (excluding delusions of reference)
- Odd beliefs or magical thinking, inconsistent with cultural norms
- Unusual perceptual experiences (such as bodily illusions)
- Suspiciousness
- Inappropriate or restricted affect
- Odd or eccentric appearance or behavior
- Few close friends or confidants
- Odd thinking or speech (eg, vague, stereotyped)
- Excessive social anxiety

Magical thinking may include:
- Belief in clairvoyance or telepathy
- Bizarre fantasies or preoccupations
- Belief in superstitions

Odd behaviors may include involvement in cults or strange religious practices

What is the differential diagnosis of schizotypal PD?

Psychotic symptoms in schizophrenia, autistic disorder, Asperger disorder, and other personality disorders

! What is a good way to distinguish between schizotypal and schizoid PD?

- For schizoid PD, think of **"Batman"**: withdrawn, no desire to interact with other people.
- For schizotypal PD, think of **"The Joker"**: outwardly strange behavior, odd beliefs.

! What is the difference between schizotypal PD and schizophrenia?

Patients with schizotypal PD are not frankly psychotic, although they can be transiently.

What is the treatment for schizotypal PD?

Psychotherapy is the treatment of choice. Short-term antipsychotic medication can be used for transient psychosis.

CLUSTER B ("WILD")

Antisocial Personality Disorder

What is the prevalence of antisocial PD?

3% is men, 1% in women

What populations and areas contain a higher incidence of antisocial PD?

More common in lower socioeconomic areas and prisons

What is the risk of antisocial PD in relatives of those afflicted with this disorder?

Five times increased risk among first-degree relatives

What other psychiatric diseases are more commonly seen among relatives of individuals with antisocial PD?

Somatization disorder and substance-related disorders

What family characteristics have been associated with the development of antisocial behavior?

Physical abuse, family discord, and a parental history of alcoholism

! **What are the *DSM-IV* diagnostic criteria for antisocial PD?**

Pattern of disregard for others and violation of the rights of others since age of 15. Patients must be **at least 18 years old** for this diagnosis; history of behavior as a child/adolescent must be consistent with **conduct disorder** (see Chapter 6). Three or more of the following should be present:

- Failure to conform to social norms by committing unlawful acts
- Deceitfulness/repeated lying/ manipulating others for personal gain
- Impulsivity/failure to plan ahead
- Irritability and aggressiveness/ repeated fights or assaults
- Recklessness and disregard for safety of self or others
- Irresponsibility/failure to sustain work or honor financial obligations
- Lack of remorse for actions

What is the differential diagnosis of antisocial PD?

Intermittent explosive disorder, substance-related disorders, manic episodes in bipolar disorder or schizoaffective disorder, and other personality disorders

! How does one distinguish antisocial PD from intermittent explosive disorder?

Individuals with intermittent explosive disorder exhibit discrete episodes of loss of control. They show little or no signs of general impulsiveness or aggressiveness between these episodes. Also, they tend to be remorseful and worried about the consequences of their actions.

! What is the difference between antisocial behavior associated with antisocial PD versus that seen with substance-related disorders?

Antisocial behavior associated with substance-related disorders occurs only in the context of disinhibition from substance intoxication or emotional lability from substance withdrawal. The behavior is not present during periods of sobriety. Patients with antisocial PD will display antisocial behaviors whether they are intoxicated or not.

In addition to the symptoms mentioned in the DSM criteria, what trait might an antisocial person display in a clinical interview?

Antisocial persons are known to be charming individuals. This attribute makes them good at manipulating others.

! What is the typical course of antisocial PD?

Onset of symptoms during childhood. Early adulthood is often complicated by drug abuse, poor academic and occupational performance, and criminal behavior. Symptoms may improve as patient ages.

How is antisocial PD treated?

Goals of treatment are to decrease impulsivity and increase the individual's conformity with societal values.

- Group and individual psychotherapies are the treatment of choice.
- "Limit-setting" (ie, refusal of acquaintances to tolerate abuse) for antisocial behaviors is often necessary.
- Pharmacotherapy can be used for symptoms of anxiety or depression.

Borderline Personality Disorder

What is the prevalence of borderline personality disorder (BPD)?

1%-2%

! Are there any gender disparities in the incidence of BPD?

Yes. Women are **twice as likely** to have borderline PD.

What psychiatric comorbidities are often seen in patients with BPD?

Mood disorders (especially depression), substance-related disorders, eating disorders, and posttraumatic stress disorder

What psychiatric diseases are more commonly seen among relatives of individuals with BPD?

BPD, antisocial PD, substance-related disorders, and mood disorders

! What percentage of patients with BPD commit suicide?

10%-15%

! What are the *DSM-IV* diagnostic criteria for BPD?

Pervasive pattern of impulsivity and **unstable relationships**, affects self-image and behaviors, present by early adulthood and in a variety of contexts. At least five of the following must be present:

- Desperate efforts to avoid real or imagined abandonment
- Unstable, intense interpersonal relationships
- Unstable self-image
- Impulsivity in at least two potentially harmful ways (eg, spending, sexual activity, substance use)
- Recurrent suicidal threats or attempts or **self-mutilation**
- Unstable mood/affect
- General feeling of emptiness
- Difficulty controlling anger
- Transient, stress-related paranoid ideation or dissociative symptoms

What is the differential diagnosis of BPD?

Mood disorders (especially bipolar disorder and cyclothymia), other personality disorders, and adolescent angst

! What is often seen in the social history of patients with BPD?

Higher rates of childhood sexual, emotional, and physical abuse

What are some defense mechanisms used by people with BPD?

Splitting, denial, projection, projective identification, acting out, and idealization. (For definitions of common defense mechanisms, see Chapter 1.)

! **What is splitting?**

The tendency to view people or events as either all good or all bad. A classic example is for a borderline patient to view one of his/her doctors as perfect and the others as bad, which can cause conflict amongst the treatment team.

What is acting out?

Performing an action to express (often unconscious) emotional conflicts. Examples are throwing a temper tantrum or behaving promiscuously.

What are "micro-psychotic" episodes?

Transient episodes in which patients may appear psychotic because of the intensity of their distress and resultant distortions. This is seen commonly in patients with BPD.

What is the typical course of BPD?

Usually chronic; some improvement in symptoms is seen with age

! **How is BPD treated?**

Goals of treatment are to improve emotional stability, sense of identity, and interpersonal relationships, and to decrease self-destructive behavior.

- Psychotherapies such as Dialectic Behavioral and Mindfulness Therapies are the treatment of choice and have been shown to help with mood/affect lability, anger control, depressive symptoms, and self-harm behavior.
- Selective serotonin reuptake inhibitors (SSRIs) and mood stabilizers (eg, Lithium) have been shown to be modestly helpful in reducing the symptoms listed above.

Where does the term "borderline" come from?

Historically, it was used to describe individuals who were considered to be on the "borderline" between neurosis and psychosis.

Histrionic Personality Disorder

Are there any gender disparities in the incidence of HPD?

Yes. It is more common in women.

What are the *DSM-IV* diagnostic criteria for HPD?

Pattern of **excessive emotionality and attention seeking**, present by early adulthood and in a variety of contexts. At least five of the following must be present:
- Uncomfortable when not the center of attention
- **Inappropriately seductive or provocative behavior**
- Uses physical appearance to draw attention to self
- Has speech that is impressionistic and lacking in detail
- Theatrical and exaggerated expression of emotion
- Easily influenced by others or situation
- Perceives relationships as more intimate than they actually are

What is the differential diagnosis of HPD?

Other personality disorders, particularly BPD and narcissistic personality disorder (NPD)

! **How does one distinguish between BPD and HPD?**

Patients with BPD are generally more depressed and suicidal than those with HPD; also, patients with HPD are generally **more functional**.

What are some common defense mechanisms used by people with HPD?

Repression, **sexualization**, regression, and somatization

How is HPD treated?

Psychotherapy is the treatment of choice. Pharmacotherapy can be used for depressive or anxious symptoms as necessary.

Narcissistic Personality Disorder

Are there any gender disparities in the incidence of NPD?

Yes. It is 1.5 times more common in men.

What are the *DSM-IV* diagnostic criteria for NPD?

Pattern of **grandiosity**, need for admiration, and lack of empathy beginning in early adulthood and present in a variety of contexts. Five or more of the following must be present:

- Exaggerated sense of self-importance
- Preoccupied with fantasies of unlimited money, success, brilliance, and so on
- Believes that he or she is "special" or unique and can associate only with other high-status individuals
- Needs excessive admiration
- Has sense of **entitlement**
- Takes advantage of others for self-gain
- Lacks empathy
- Envious of others or believes others are envious of him or her
- Arrogant or haughty

What is the differential diagnosis of NPD?

Other personality disorders, particularly antisocial and BPDs, and manic or hypomanic episodes

How does one distinguish between antisocial PD and NPD?

Both types of patients exploit others, but the goal of NPD patients is status and recognition, while antisocial PD patients desire material gain or simply the subjugation of others.

What is "entitlement"?

Entitlement is a stable and pervasive sense that one deserves more than others.

What are some common defense mechanisms used by people with NPD?

Idealization (of themselves) and devaluation (of other people)

What is the typical course of NPD?

Chronic course; higher incidence of depression and midlife crises since these patients put such a high value on youth and power

How is NPD treated?

Psychotherapy is the treatment of choice. Antidepressants or lithium can be used as needed for comorbid mood disorders.

CLUSTER C ("WORRIED")

Avoidant Personality Disorder

! What are the *DSM-IV* diagnostic criteria for avoidant PD?

Pattern of **social inhibition,** hypersensitivity and feelings of inadequacy since early adulthood, with at least four of the following:

- Avoids occupation that involves interpersonal contact due to a **fear of criticism or rejection**
- Unwilling to interact unless certain of being liked
- Cautious of interpersonal relationships
- Preoccupied with being criticized or rejected in social situations
- Inhibited in new social situations because he or she feels inadequate
- Believes he or she is socially inept and inferior
- Reluctant to engage in new activities for fear of embarrassment

What is the differential diagnosis of avoidant PD?

Social anxiety disorder, schizoid PD, dependent PD, and other personality disorders

! How does one distinguish between social anxiety disorder and avoidant PD?

Although both disorders involve fear and avoidance of social situations, avoidant PD is an overall fear of **rejection** and affects many areas of life, while social anxiety disorder is a fear of **embarrassment** in a particular setting. (See Chapter 2 for details)

! How does one distinguish between schizoid PD and avoidant PD?

Patients with avoidant PD desire companionship but fear being rejected, whereas patients with schizoid PD have no desire for companionship.

How is avoidant PD treated?

- Psychotherapy, including assertiveness training, is the treatment of choice.
- Anxiolytics (eg, beta-blockers) can be used for symptoms of anxiety.
- Antidepressants can be used for depressive symptoms.

Dependent Personality Disorder

Are there any gender disparities in the incidence of DPD?

Yes. Women are more likely to have DPD.

What are the *DSM-IV* diagnostic criteria for DPD?

Pattern of **submissive and clinging** behavior due to excessive need to be taken care of. At least five of the following must be present:

- Difficulty making everyday decisions without reassurance from others
- Needs others to assume responsibilities for most areas of his or her life
- Cannot express disagreement because of fear of loss of approval
- Difficulty initiating projects because of lack of self-confidence
- Goes to excessive lengths to obtain support from others
- Feels helpless when alone
- **Urgently seeks another relationship when one ends**
- Preoccupied with fears of being left to take care of self

What is the differential diagnosis of DPD?

Disability resulting from another medical or psychiatric disorder, and other personality disorders, especially avoidant, borderline, and histrionic PD

How does one distinguish between disabled persons and DPD patients?

Many people with debilitating illnesses can develop dependent traits. However, to be diagnosed with DPD, the features described above must manifest before early adulthood.

! How does one distinguish between dependent PD and avoidant PD?

Avoidant PD patients are slow to get involved in relationships, whereas dependent PD patients actively and aggressively seek out relationships.

How are the relationships of patients with DPD different from those with BPD and HPD?

DPD patients generally have a long-lasting relationship with the person on whom they are dependent. BPD and HPD patients are often unable to maintain long-lasting relationships.

How is DPD treated?

- Psychotherapy and cognitive-behavioral therapy are effective. The therapist must be careful not to allow the patient to become too dependent on the doctor-patient relationship.
- Pharmacotherapy can be used for symptoms of depression or anxiety.

Obsessive-Compulsive Personality Disorder

Are there any gender disparities in the incidence of OCPD?

Men are nearly twice as likely to have OCPD.

What is the risk of OCPD in relatives of those afflicted with this disorder?

Increased incidence in first-degree relatives

! **What are the *DSM-IV* diagnostic criteria for OCPD?**

Pattern of **preoccupation with orderliness, control, and perfectionism** at the expense of efficiency, present by early adulthood and in a variety of contexts. At least four of the following must be present:

- Preoccupation with details, rules, lists, and organization such that the major point of the activity is lost
- Perfectionism that is detrimental to completion of task
- Excessive devotion to work
- Excessive conscientiousness and scrupulousness about morals and ethics
- Will not delegate tasks
- Unable to discard worthless objects
- Miserly
- Rigid and stubborn

What is the differential diagnosis of OCPD?

Obsessive-compulsive disorder and other personality disorders, especially NPD and PPD

! **How does one distinguish between obsessive-compulsive disorder and OCPD?**

Patients with OCPD do not have the recurrent obsessions and compulsions that are present in obsessive-compulsive disorder, and their symptoms are **ego-syntonic**, meaning that they may not be aware that they have a problem. Symptoms in obsessive-compulsive disorder are **ego-dystonic**, meaning that they cause the patient distress.

What are some common defense mechanisms used by people with OCPD?

Intellectualization, rationalization, isolation of affect, reaction formation, displacement, and undoing. OCPD patients often have difficulty recognizing or expressing their own anger, and they fear losing control of it; thus, they use defense mechanisms such as reaction formation and displacement of anger.

What is the prime issue for OCPD patients in their interpersonal relationships?

Control. OCPD patients seek to remain in control of themselves and to control those around them.

How is OCPD treated?

- Psychotherapy is the treatment of choice. Group therapy and behavioral therapy can also be useful.
- Pharmacotherapy can be used for associated symptoms as necessary.

Personality Disorder Not Otherwise Specified

What are the *DSM-IV* diagnostic criteria of personality disorder not otherwise specified (PD NOS)?

This category is for disorders of personality functioning that do not meet criteria for any specific personality disorder. An example is the presence of features of more than one specific personality disorder that do not meet the full criteria for any one personality disorder ("mixed personality"), but that together cause clinically significant distress or impairment in one or more important areas of functioning (eg, social or occupational).

What are some examples of PD NOS?

Depressive personality disorder and passive-aggressive personality disorder

CLINICAL VIGNETTES

A 46-year-old woman lives alone in a dilapidated house in a residential neighborhood. She spends most of her time collecting items from other people's trash. According to her neighbors, she refers to these items as her "antique collection." Despite having lived in the neighborhood for many years, she does not have any friends and mostly keeps to herself. When a neighbor approached her recently and criticized the condition of her house, the woman seemed unfazed. What is the likely diagnosis?

Schizoid personality disorder; this disorder involves a pattern of voluntary social withdrawal and restricted range of emotional expression, beginning by early adulthood and present in a variety of contexts. Patients with this disorder are typically indifferent to criticism or praise.

A 35-year-old man is described by his acquaintances as something of an "odd duck." A few years ago he was convinced that his neighbors were conspiring against him, but he no longer thinks that this is true. He has strewn an assortment of dolls on his front lawn, stating that he believes that they will bring him good luck. Once in a while, he is seen walking from house to house in his neighborhood, seeking to enlist members for a "new age" religion that he claims to have founded. What is the likely diagnosis?

Schizotypal personality disorder; this disorder involves a pattern of social deficits marked by eccentric behavior, cognitive or perceptual distortions, and discomfort with close relationships, beginning by early adulthood and present in a variety of contexts. Patients with this disorder may display magical thinking and bizarre fantasies. Schizotypal personality disorder must be distinguished from schizophrenia, in which patients are frankly psychotic.

A 35-year-old woman presents to her primary care doctor with her boyfriend of 6 months. She complains that since the beginning of their relationship, her boyfriend has become increasingly helpless. She claims that he is unable to make simple, everyday decisions without her help, and is constantly seeking her support and approval. When asked for his opinion, the boyfriend seems afraid to disagree with her. After further questioning of the man, the physician discovers that he has been in one relationship after another for all of his adult life. What is the likely diagnosis of this man?

Dependent personality disorder; this disorder involves a pattern of submissive and clinging behavior due to excessive need to be taken care of. Common features of this disorder include an inability to express disagreement because of fear of loss of approval and the urgent seeking of another relationship once one ends.

A 37-year-old man is arrested for auto theft. According to his record, he has had five other arrests since the age of 13, for offenses ranging from aggravated assault to vandalism. He also has a history of aggressiveness toward authority and general recklessness. When asked if he feels bad about his actions, he replies "Why should I?" What is the likely diagnosis?

Antisocial personality disorder; this disorder involves a pattern of disregard for others and violation of the rights of others since age of 15. Patients with this disorder tend to lack remorse for their actions.

A 43-year-old woman presents to her primary care doctor for a regular checkup. She appears to be out of breath and states that she "almost died a few times" on the way to her doctor's office. Her doctor notices that she answers his questions in much exaggerated terms, but that her answers lack precise detail. Moreover, her speech is provocative and flirtatious. When the doctor excuses himself to answer a telephone call, the patient grows irate, claiming that his job is to pay attention to her. What is the likely diagnosis?

Histrionic personality disorder; this disorder involves a pattern of excessive emotionality and attention seeking, present by early adulthood and in a variety of contexts. Patients with this disorder often engage in inappropriately seductive or provocative behavior to draw attention to themselves.

A 29-year-old woman has begun to alienate her coworkers with her behavior. She continually states that no one else is able to meet her standards of excellence, and she constantly berates her colleagues to work harder. Despite her beliefs about the high quality of her work, she frequently misses deadlines, as she spends most of her time focusing on the minor, often irrelevant details of projects. She is known to brag about her great "relationship with God," and she is quick to judge others on what she perceives as their "moral shortcomings." What is the likely diagnosis?

Obsessive-compulsive personality disorder; this disorder involves a pattern of preoccupation with orderliness, control, and perfectionism at the expense of efficiency, present by early adulthood and in a variety of contexts. Patients with this disorder often exhibit excessive conscientiousness and scrupulousness about morals and ethics. Obsessive-compulsive personality disorder must be distinguished from obsessive-compulsive disorder, in which patients have recurrent obsessions and compulsions that cause them distress.

A 39-year-old man is admitted to the ER after a minor automobile accident. He refuses to let the residents treat him, claiming that only the "chief of the department" is good enough for him. When told that the chief is not available at the moment, he requests a phone, saying that he will "call in some favors." He becomes enraged when a nurse tells him that all of the phones are currently being used; he yells "Can't you see I deserve a phone more than anyone else in here!?" What is the likely diagnosis?

Narcissistic personality disorder; this disorder involves a pattern of grandiosity, need for admiration, and lack of empathy beginning in early adulthood and present in a variety of contexts.

A 40-year-old woman is known by her colleagues as an extremely private person. She seems generally mistrustful of those around her and is reluctant to confide in anyone. Every now and again she is heard accusing various coworkers of conspiring against her. One coworker relates a story in which the president of the company asked her what she was doing after work; in response, she became very fearful and demanded to know why anyone needed to know such information. What is the likely diagnosis? What other disorder is this woman at risk for?

Paranoid personality disorder. Increased risk for paranoid schizophrenia; this disorder involves a general distrust of others, beginning by early adulthood and present in a variety of contexts. Patients with this disorder are at elevated risk for developing schizophrenia. Paranoid personality disorder must be distinguished from paranoid schizophrenia, in which patients have fixed delusions and are frankly psychotic.

A 38-year-old woman presents to her primary care doctor with the complaint that she has become very lonely. She appears very shy before the doctor and admits to a desire to join new social clubs, but she is "petrified" that people will think that she "isn't cool." She reports that she recently quit her job as a receptionist because having to greet people every day became too stressful, as she is convinced that she always "makes a bad first impression." However, she insists to her physician that she would really like to make some new friends. What is the likely diagnosis?

Avoidant personality disorder; this disorder involves a pattern of social inhibition, hypersensitivity, and feelings of inadequacy since early adulthood. Patients with this disorder are typically preoccupied with being criticized or rejected in social situations.

A 46-year-old woman begins psychotherapy stating that she feels a "void" in her life. She reports having attempted suicide a few times in the past, and she has seen various psychiatrists throughout her life. She describes engaging in a number of impulsive behaviors, particularly those involving promiscuity. She states that she is always "demanding" of her psychiatrists, and that these high standards have led her to terminate therapy in a number of cases. Throughout the course of the interview, the patient describes herself in a variety of ways, often contradicting herself. At one point she says that she is quite liberal; at another moment, she claims to be very conservative. She ends the interview by stating that she is "desperate" to figure out what her goals in life should be. What is the likely diagnosis, and what is a common finding in the past history of patients with this diagnosis?

Borderline personality disorder; this disorder involves a pervasive pattern of impulsivity and unstable relationships, affects self-image and behaviors, present by early adulthood and in a variety of contexts. Research has documented a high frequency of neglect, abandonment, physical abuse, and sexual abuse in the history of individuals with this disorder.

A 40-year-old woman presents to the ER after slashing her wrists. This is the fifth time in her life that she has made a suicidal gesture, and she explains that death would be a way for her to escape the "emptiness" that plagues her. Her medical records indicate that she has seen many psychiatrists in the past. When asked why she has changed psychiatrists so many times, she states that they abandoned her and that it was not her fault. She goes on to comment that the doctors in the ER have treated her "perfectly," while the nursing staff has been "the worst" she has ever seen. What defense mechanism does this patient display? What treatment would be most effective for her illness?

Splitting. Treat with psychotherapy; the patient uses "splitting," a complex defense mechanism in which others are seen as either all good (and thus caring, rescuing sources of strength) or all bad (and thus to blame for all one's own misery). She suffers from borderline personality disorder, which involves a pervasive pattern of impulsivity and unstable relationships, affects self-image and behaviors, present by early adulthood and in a variety of contexts. The treatment of choice is psychotherapy.

CHAPTER 6

Childhood Disorders

What are the three components of the psychiatric assessment of a child?

1. Consideration of child's stage of development
2. Attention to and observation of family structure and dynamics
3. Evaluation for normative age-appropriate behavior

How do children express emotion differently than adults?

Children tend to express emotion more concretely, whereas adults tend to express emotion abstractly.

How does the different manner in which children express emotion change the approach to their psychiatric evaluation?

Questions are asked about the absence or presence of manifestations of emotion rather than of the emotion itself. For example, "Do you feel like screaming?" rather than "Are you angry?"

Besides questioning, what other methods are employed by child psychiatrists in evaluation?

Roleplaying with games, toys, dolls, or drawing

What psychological test is most widely used to assess children of school age?

Wechsler Intelligence Scale for Children-Revised (WISC-R)

What score is derived from the WISC-R?

IQ or intelligence quotient representing a verbal score and a performance score

What psychological test is most widely used to assess very young children?

Stanford-Binet

How is IQ defined?

Mental age divided by chronologic age and multiplied by 100

MENTAL RETARDATION

What is the primary disturbance in mental retardation?	Intelligence is subnormal, leading to difficulties in adaptive functioning.
! **What IQ score is required for the diagnosis of mental retardation?**	Less than 70

Epidemiology and Etiology

What is the prevalence of mental retardation in the population?	1%-2%
What gender presents with mental retardation more frequently?	2:1 male to female ratio
Does the incidence of mental retardation show any relationship to socioeconomic status?	Milder forms can be associated with low socioeconomic status, whereas more severe forms show no association.
In the mentally retarded population, what degree of mental retardation is most prevalent?	85% of mental retardation is graded as "mild."
What degree of mental retardation is associated with general medical conditions?	Severe retardation
! **What is the most common cause of mental retardation?**	Down syndrome (trisomy 21)
! **What is the most common cause of inherited mental retardation?**	Fragile X syndrome

Diagnosis

How may children present with mental retardation?	Failure or delay in meeting developmental milestones, poor intellectual functioning
! **What physical examination findings are associated with Down syndrome?**	Single horizontal palmar crease, almond-shaped eyes, flat hypoplastic face with short nose, prominent epicanthic skin folds, small, low-set ears, protruding tongue

What three characteristics must be present to make the diagnosis of mental retardation?

1. Onset before age 18
2. IQ less than 70
3. Impaired adaptation to environments such as home, work, social

What tests are indicated in patients suspected of having mental retardation?

IQ tests, electroencephalogram, computed tomography (CT), or magnetic resonance imaging (MRI) in addition to metabolic or genetic testing specific for suspected underlying disorders

What does the differential diagnosis for mental retardation include?

Attention deficit hyperactivity disorder (ADHD), depression, learning disorders, schizophrenia, seizure disorder, pervasive developmental disorder (PDD)

What percentage of mentally retarded children has comorbid ADHD?

10%-20%

LEARNING DISORDERS

! **What defines learning disorders?**

Academic achievement in specific areas below the level expected by a child's chronologic age, measured intelligence, and age-appropriate education

Name the three learning disorders identified by the *DSM-IV (Diagnostic and Statistical Manual of Mental Disorders, Fourth Edition).*

1. Mathematics disorder
2. Reading disorder
3. Disorder of written expression

Epidemiology and Etiology

What is the prevalence of learning disorders in school-age children?

Ranges from 2% to 10%

What gender presents with learning disorders more frequently?

Up to 4:1 male to female ratio

Can learning disorders be familial?

Yes

What are other postulated causes of learning disorders?

- Focal cerebral injury
- Neurodevelopmental defect

! What are some substance-induced conditions that are associated with learning disorders?

Lead poisoning and fetal alcohol syndrome

Diagnosis

How can learning disorders be diagnosed?

Specific intelligence and achievement testing

When are most learning disorders diagnosed?

Between first and fifth grade of elementary school

! What is the differential diagnosis for learning disorders?

- External factors such as socioeconomic disadvantages, poor schooling, or language barriers
- Medical factors such as hearing or vision impairment
- Global functioning factors such as communication disorders, mental retardation, PDDs

How does dyslexia present?

Difficulty in reading especially in comprehension, word order, and letter sequence in children of normal IQ

What difficulties result from dyslexia?

Problems with spelling and verbal language

Treatment

How can learning disorders be treated?

Special individualized education to teach material in the most effective manner in addition to remediation for the specific learning disorder

Is dyslexia self-limited in children?

No, difficulties persist into adulthood

AUTISTIC DISORDER

To what spectrum of disorders does autistic disorder belong?

Pervasive Developmental Disorders (PPD). Other examples of PDD are Asperger disorder, Rett disorder, and childhood disintegrative disorder.

! **What is the triad of findings in autistic disorder?**	1. Impaired social interactions 2. Impaired communication skills 3. Highly limited set of activities and interests; often object oriented and repetitive

Epidemiology and Etiology

What is the incidence of autistic disorder?	2-5 children per 10,000 live births
! **What gender presents with autistic disorder more frequently?**	Up to 5:1 male to female ratio
Is autistic disorder familial?	Yes: incomplete penetrance is implicated by genetic studies.
Can autistic disorder result from poor or conflicting parenting styles?	No. Original psychodynamic theory offered this idea; however, it was later disproved.
Can autism be caused by vaccine administration?	No.
What other disorders have been associated with autistic disorder?	Tuberous sclerosis, fragile X, phenylketonuria (PKU), maternal rubella, perinatal anoxia, encephalitis

Diagnosis

! **What is the most frequent initial disturbance noted in patients with autistic disorder?**	Impairment in social interactions resulting in lack of peer relationships and poor recognition or response to social cues
! **What are examples of social impairment that satisfy *DSM-IV* criteria for autistic disorder?**	• Poor eye contact • Failure to develop a social smile • Lack of facial expression • Unwillingness to make friends • Not sharing or pointing out objects of enjoyment
! **What are examples of impairment in communication that satisfy *DSM-IV* criteria for autistic disorder?**	• Markedly slowed language development • Difficulty initiating or maintaining conversation • Limited or repetitive use of vocabulary • Abnormal alterations in pitch, intonation, rate, rhythm, or stress

! What are examples of behaviors and interests that satisfy *DSM-IV* criteria for autistic disorder?

- *Restrictive:* Knowledge is narrow and limited to one or few topics or attention is focused on parts of objects.
- *Repetitive:* Specific motor activity is stereotyped and becomes a preoccupation such as hand flapping.
- *Inflexible:* Certain activities must be conducted at the same time or in the same manner each day and become ritualistic.

! What time course of delays satisfies *DSM-IV* criteria for autistic disorder?

Delays in social interaction, communication, or symbolic or imaginative play must begin before the age of 3.

! What percentage of children with autistic disorder has comorbid seizures?

25%

! What percentage of children with autistic disorder has mental retardation?

75%

What does the differential diagnosis of autistic disorder include?

Childhood psychosis, congenital deafness or blindness, language disorders, mental retardation

At what age does autistic disorder usually become evident?

2 or 3 years of age

What is selective mutism?

The inability to speak in certain situations. Patients function normally in other areas of behavior and learning, though appear withdrawn and some are unable to participate in group activities. As an example, a child may be completely silent at school, for years at a time, but speak quite freely or even excessively at home.

How can selective mutism be distinguished from other childhood disorders?

Consistent failure to speak in a **specific social situation** despite talking in other situations is not a characteristic of other disorders such as autism or separation anxiety disorder.

Treatment

What is the prognosis for autistic disorder?

The disorder is chronic and lifelong with no cure presently.

What is the primary goal in managing autistic disorder?

Developing behavioral management techniques

What are the goals of behavioral management techniques?

Reducing repetitive and inflexible behaviors while improving social and communicative functioning

What pharmacologic treatment is indicated for autistic disorder?

- Anticonvulsants for comorbid seizures
- Neuroleptics in low doses to decrease aggression
- Mood stabilizers and antidepressants have also been used

ASPERGER DISORDER

What is Asperger disorder?

A PDD characterized by impaired social interaction and restricted interests and activities

How is Asperger disorder similar to autism?

Both disorders share qualitative impairments in social interaction and a restricted range of interests and activities.

! **How do the *DSM-IV* criteria for Asperger disorder differ from autism?**

Asperger disorder is always characterized by normal language and cognitive development.

RETT DISORDER

What is Rett disorder?

A PDD in which multiple deficits arise following a relatively normal birth and initial period of development

! **What is the major difference between autistic disorder and Rett disorder?**

Rett disorder is always characterized by an initial period of normal development.

In which gender does Rett disorder almost exclusively occur?

Female because the disorder is X-linked thus resulting in fatal outcome in males

What is the etiology of Rett disorder?

Genetic; mosaic defect at chromosomal site Xq28 involving the MECP2 gene

! **What are the *DSM-IV* criteria for diagnosis of Rett disorder?**

1. Normal prenatal and perinatal development
2. Normal psychomotor development for at least **5 months** after birth
3. Normal head circumference at birth
4. Onset of deficits following the initially normal period of development that must include:
   a. Deceleration of head growth between 5 and 48 months
   b. **Loss of hand coordination between 5 and 30 months**
   c. **Onset of unusual, repetitive hand movements (such as hand wringing)**
   d. Loss of social engagement
   e. Impairments in coordination of gait or trunk movements
   f. Severe retardation

CHILDHOOD DISINTEGRATIVE DISORDER

! **What *DSM-IV* criteria characterize childhood disintegrative disorder?**

Loss of previously acquired skills and onset of autistic symptoms following a 2-year period of normal development

In what gender is childhood disintegrative disorder more common?

Four to eight times more common in males

! **What are the two major differences between childhood disintegrative disorder and Rett disorder?**

1. *Gender:* Rett disorder affects females, whereas childhood disintegrative disorder is more common in males
2. *Duration of preceding normal period of development:* Rett disorder—5 months versus childhood disintegrative disorder—2 years

ATTENTION DEFICIT HYPERACTIVITY DISORDER

What behaviors are implicated in ADHD?

- Overactivity, cannot sit still
- Poor impulse control
- Inattention
- Distractibility
- Disruptive in class

How is the pattern of such behaviors characterized and differentiated from individuals without ADHD?

- Persistent
- Dysfunctional

Epidemiology and Etiology

What is the prevalence of ADHD in school-age children?

3%-5%

What gender presents with ADHD more frequently?

4:1 male to female ratio in the general population, 9:1 male to female ratio in clinical settings such as primary care or psychiatric outpatient visits

What accounts for the difference in gender presentation between general and clinical populations?

Males are more likely to be identified and referred to clinic.

Does ADHD show a familial pattern?

Yes

What disorders are more common in families who have a child diagnosed with ADHD?

Antisocial personality disorders, mood disorders (especially bipolar disorder), substance use disorders, and learning disorders

Diagnosis

! **Name the *DSM-IV* criteria required for the diagnosis of ADHD.**

- Onset of inattentive, hyperactive, or impulsive symptoms before age 7
- Symptoms must be present in two or more settings, usually school and home
- Duration of symptoms exceeds 6 months

! **If ADHD symptoms are present in only one setting, what cause is suggested?**

Environmental or psychodynamic

How may children present with ADHD?

- Stay up late
- Wake up early
- Most time is spent in a hyperactive or impulsive state
- May cause damage or be unmanageable around the house
- Exhibit difficulty following directions
- Forget assignments or school supplies
- Do not wait for their turn to be called on in class
- Difficulty sustaining attention during tests
- Difficulty staying in his/her seat

What complications may result if this behavior is not correctly identified as ADHD?

Children may be viewed as troublemakers and receive negative treatment. Teachers may avoid giving them educational attention because of the effort required for discipline. As a result, these children may lag behind the others academically and socially.

What aspects of the history, physical examination, and diagnostic testing are important in making the diagnosis of ADHD?

- History obtained from parents and teachers
- Observation of behavior at school and at home
- Complete neurologic examination
- Tests of attention such as completing puzzles and sequential or ordered tasks
- Tests to rule out learning disorders, including IQ testing

What is the main differential diagnosis for the hyperactive symptoms of ADHD?

Age-appropriate behaviors in active children; mania

What are the main differential diagnoses for the inattentive symptoms of ADHD?

- Mismatch between IQ and level of stimulation from the child's environment
- Outright refusal to perform a task in oppositional defiant disorder
- Mood disorders
- Medication side effects
- Psychotic disorders
- PDD

! How can the inattentiveness in children with mood disorders be differentiated from children with ADHD?

- Inattentiveness after the age of 7 often implies mood disorders.
- School adjustment in children with mood disorders is complicated by psychosocial factors in excess of inattention and disruptive behavior.

How would one distinguish between ADHD and mania?

Children with ADHD often suffer from low self-esteem, while children with mania are more likely to be euphoric. Pressured speech, distractibility, motoric overactivity, and impulsivity are seen in both disorders.

Treatment

What are the goals in treatment of ADHD?

Improve performance in the classroom, improve self-esteem, prevent behavioral complications

What pharmacologic class is used with greatest benefit in children with ADHD?

Psychostimulants

! **What drugs are considered first line to treat ADHD?**

Short- and intermediate-acting, and extended release methylphenidate (Ritalin, Concerta) and short- and intermediate-acting, and extended release dextroamphetamine (Dexedrine, Adderall)

What drugs are considered second line to treat ADHD?

Antidepressants, such as tricyclics (eg, imipramine and desipramine) and bupropion (Wellbutrin), and the norepinephrine reuptake inhibitor atomoxetine (Stratterra)

What dosing strategy is employed when using psychostimulants in children?

- Using the smallest effective dose
- Limiting use of medication to periods when it is needed most

Does the use of stimulants in children with ADHD lead to drug abuse or addiction in adulthood?

No

In what percentage of children with ADHD do symptoms persist into adulthood?

30%

How is the treatment of ADHD different in mentally retarded children?

It is not. Stimulants are equally effective in mentally retarded individuals.

In addition to pharmacologic treatment, what other modalities are used in managing ADHD?

Behavioral strategies such as positive reinforcement for appropriate behaviors and task completion, limit setting, and tailoring environmental stimulation to manageable levels

CONDUCT DISORDER

What is conduct disorder?

Persistent pattern of repeatedly violating societal norms, rules, or the rights of others

What are examples of behavior seen in conduct disorder?

Destroying property, aggression against people or animals, theft, running away

! **What personality disorder in adults is equivalent to conduct disorder in children?**

Antisocial personality disorder

Etiology and Epidemiology

In what percentage of school-age children does conduct disorder occur?

3%-7%

! **What gender presents with conduct disorder more frequently?**

9:1 male to female ratio

Diagnosis

! **What are the *DSM-IV* diagnostic criteria for conduct disorder?**

- Persistent pattern of behavior that violates societal norms or the basic rights of people or animals as manifest by three or more of the following:
    - Violence
    - Rape
    - Vandalism
    - Fire setting
    - Lying
    - Theft
    - Truancy
- Duration of such behavior for at least 1 year

What features or diagnoses are associated with conduct disorder?

Dysfunctional family, learning disorders, ADHD, physical injuries as a result of fighting, substance abuse, inability to keep a job, failing school

Treatment

What is the treatment for conduct disorder?	Individual and family therapy; behavioral techniques such as limit setting; occasionally removal of the child from home environment and placement in foster care; role modeling; moral instruction; structured living settings
! What percentage of children with conduct disorder progress to antisocial personality disorder as adults?	25%-40%
! What disorders are present in adulthood among children and adolescents with conduct disorder?	Antisocial personality disorder, somatoform disorders, depression, substance abuse

OPPOSITIONAL DEFIANT DISORDER

What is oppositional defiant disorder?	A disorder of childhood or adolescence characterized by a recurrent pattern of negativistic, hostile, and disobedient behavior toward authority figures
! How does oppositional defiant disorder differ from conduct disorder?	• Annoying, disruptive, argumentative, and disobedient behavior toward authority • Usually without destructive and aggressive behaviors • Sense of empathy for others is preserved • Maintain respect for other people's rights
In what gender does oppositional defiant disorder more frequently present?	Male
What are children with oppositional defiant disorder at risk for?	Developing conduct disorder

TOURETTE DISORDER

! **What characterizes Tourette disorder?**
Multiple, involuntary, and uncontrollable motor and vocal tics

What is a "tic"?
Sudden, swift, repetitive, arrhythmic, and stereotyped movement or vocalization. A tic can be actively suppressed but when performed bring about a sense of relief to the patient.

Epidemiology and Etiology

What gender presents with Tourette disorder more frequently?
3:1 male to female ratio

Does Tourette disorder show any familial pattern?
Yes

What disorders are most frequently associated with Tourette disorder?
Obsessive-compulsive disorder and ADHD

What is PANDAS?
Pediatric
Autoimmune
Neuropsychiatric
Disorders
Associated with
Streptococcal Infection

What is the hypothetical relationship between PANDAS and Tourette disorder?
Some cases of Tourette disorder (as well as obsessive-compulsive disorder) may be caused by an autoimmune reaction following infection by group A beta-hemolytic streptococcal infection.

Diagnosis

What is the typical age of onset of Tourette disorder?
Before age 18

! **What are the *DSM-IV* criteria for diagnosis of Tourette disorder?**
- 12 months minimum duration
- 3 months longest interval allowed without tics
- Tics during active phase can be motor only or vocal only
- Motor and vocal tics must occur together at some point

How can vocal tics in Tourette disorder be characterized?

Loud barking, grunting, or shouting words

What is coprolalia?

Involuntary utterances of obscene or vulgar words

How can motor tics in Tourette disorder be characterized?

Facial grimacing, tongue protrusion, snorting, blinking, extremity jerking

How do patients with Tourette disorder typically describe their control of vocal tics?

They are aware of their occurrence and admit to a sense of fleeting control over the tics that is overcome by an irresistible urge or compulsion to say them

What does the differential diagnosis of Tourette disorder include?

Wilson disease, Huntington disease, seizure disorder, extrapyramidal symptoms secondary to antipsychotic medication

What is a feature of Tourette disorder that distinguishes it from other hyperkinetic motor disorders?

Ability of patients to temporarily suppress their tics

Treatment

! **What is the pharmacologic treatment of Tourette disorder?**

- Atypical or typical antipsychotic agents (risperidone (Risperdal), ziprasidone (Geodon), haloperidol (Haldol), pimozide (Orap), and fluphenazine (Prolixin))
- Alpha-adrenergic agents (guanfacine, clonidine)

! **What medications are preferred to treat Tourette disorder?**

Antipsychotics. However, although other agents such as clonidine have less efficacy, they are often used due to their more favorable side effect profile.

What factors limit the use of clonidine in the treatment of Tourette disorder?

1. Lower blood pressure
2. Variable efficacy
3. May take longer to attain initial therapeutic effect over tics as compared to antipsychotic agents

What is the behavioral treatment of Tourette disorder?

While pharmacological treatment is reserved for more severe symptoms, other types of treatments (education, supportive psychotherapy) may help avoid or improve symptoms of depression or social isolation, minimize the negative social consequences of tics, and improve supportive family functioning.

NOCTURNAL ENURESIS

What is nocturnal enuresis?	Pattern of involuntary or intentional voiding of urine into bed or clothes **after age 5**, occurring at night

Etiology and Epidemiology

Is there a familial pattern to enuresis?	Yes, a history of enuresis in first-degree relatives is found in 75% of these children.
What conditions are associated with nocturnal enuresis in children?	Adjustment disorder, anxiety, oppositional defiant disorder, ADHD
What does nocturnal enuresis in adolescents imply?	Possibly, in some cases, a greater degree of underlying psychopathology

Diagnosis

! **After what age can the diagnosis of nocturnal enuresis be made?**	5 years old
When does enuresis occur in relation to onset of sleep?	In most cases 30 minutes to 3 hours after falling asleep
! **What is the frequency of enuresis that satisfies *DSM-IV* diagnostic criteria?**	At least twice a week for at least 3 consecutive months or it must cause marked impairment or distress

Treatment

! **What is the treatment for nocturnal enuresis?**	Behavior modification, psychotherapy for associated psychopathology, low doses of tricyclic antidepressants (eg, **imipramine**), desmopressin (DDAVP)
Upon resolution of enuresis what other aspects of the child's life are improved?	• Improved self-esteem • More confident social interactions

SEPARATION ANXIETY DISORDER

How does this disorder manifest in children?	Distress upon separating the child from his or her caregiver

Etiology and Epidemiology

What gender more commonly presents with separation anxiety disorder?	Male
What environmental or psychosocial aspects of a child's life may predispose him or her to separation anxiety disorder?	• Traumatic separation • Very close knit family dynamic at baseline • Mimicking of exaggerated anxiety about separation modeled by parent
What is the postulated underlying fear in the child that drives the distress in separation anxiety disorder?	Fear of harm to oneself or to loved ones

Diagnosis

! **What are symptoms of distress in separation anxiety disorder?**	• Refusal to go to school or to sleep alone • Somatic symptoms such as belly ache, head ache • Crying or screaming when being physically separated • Can progress to full-blown panic attacks
! **At what age is this behavior considered pathologic?**	• Age 1-3, normal behavior • After 3 years old, pathologic

Treatment

What type of therapy is most effective in the treatment of separation anxiety disorder?	Behavioral psychotherapy
What specific psychotherapeutic techniques are used to treat separation anxiety disorder?	Systematic desensitization and operant conditioning

When is pharmacotherapy considered in the treatment of separation anxiety disorder?

When panic is associated with separation and not entirely responsive to behavioral therapy, such as when the child is too anxious to tolerate separation or therapy

What pharmacologic agents are used in the treatment of separation anxiety disorder?

Selective serotonin reuptake inhibitors (SSRIs) or benzodiazepines

SOCIAL PHOBIA IN CHILDHOOD

What disorder did social phobia in childhood replace in *DSM-IV*?

Avoidant disorder of childhood

! **How does social phobia manifest in childhood?**

Excessive shyness and avoidance of interactions with people unfamiliar to the child after 2.5 years of age

! **Prior to 2.5 years of age, what are these symptoms considered?**

Stranger anxiety, normal developmental phenomenon

What are the complications of social phobia in childhood?

Disruption of normal psychosocial, psychosexual, self-confidence, and self-esteem development

What type of therapy is most effective in the treatment of social phobia in childhood?

Cognitive-behavioral psychotherapy with the goal of developing assertiveness

What may result from unsuccessful or ineffective treatment of social phobia in childhood?

Persistence into adulthood resulting in isolation, depression, and lack of normal social bonds

GENERALIZED ANXIETY DISORDER IN CHILDHOOD

How does generalized anxiety disorder present in children?

Excessive worry about past behavior, future events, or their own competence

What factors predispose children to generalized anxiety disorder?

- Birth order (oldest at most risk)
- Family dynamic of high performance expectations on the child
- Upper socioeconomic background
- Small family

How may children with generalized anxiety disorder behave when they are excessively anxious?

They may exhibit nervous habits, somatic complaints, seeking of reassurance or approval, and difficulty sleeping.

What is the treatment for generalized anxiety disorder in childhood?

Psychotherapy and occasionally SSRIs or benzodiazepines

CLINICAL VIGNETTES

A 5-year-old girl presents to her family physician with her parents who have been concerned that she is not progressing like the other children around her. She has not yet been toilet trained. She has difficulty writing her name, learning the alphabet, and dressing herself. Her speech is slightly difficult to understand. Her mother had limited prenatal care. IQ testing of the child was performed and calculated to be 50. The physician scheduled an MRI and ordered several metabolic and genetic tests. What is the most common cause of mental retardation? What is the most common cause of inherited mental retardation?

Down syndrome, Fragile X syndrome; the diagnosis of mental retardation is characterized by IQ less than or equal to 70, onset before age 18, and impaired adaptation to environments such as home or work. Down syndrome (trisomy 21) is the most common cause of mental retardation, whereas Fragile X syndrome is the most common cause of inherited mental retardation. Other causes include inborn errors of metabolism, maternal diabetes, early childhood head injuries, rubella, substance abuse, toxemia, and social deprivation.

A 15-year-old boy is finally brought to the physician by his foster mother after repeated requests from his school because of bad behavior. For the last year the boy has been starting fights at school, spray painting the bathroom walls with graffiti, stealing money from other students' lockers, and skipping school. Two years ago he was arrested by the police for setting fire to a neighbor's garage. He is failing all of his classes and his teachers suspect that he is using illicit drugs. What disorder may develop in persons with this disorder when they reach adulthood?

Patients with conduct disorder may develop antisocial personality disorder, somatoform disorders, depression, or substance abuse; for more than a year, this boy has exhibited a persistent pattern of behavior that violates the basic rights of people or animals or violates societal norms including violence, rape, vandalism, fire setting, theft, or truancy. This behavior is diagnostic of conduct disorder. Oppositional defiant disorder is less severe without destructive and aggressive behaviors characterized primarily by annoying, disruptive, and disobedient behavior toward authority. If the boy was older than 18, this disorder would be antisocial personality disorder. Twenty-five to forty percent of children with conduct disorder progress to antisocial personality disorder in adulthood.

An 8-year-old girl presents to her physician because she has been having trouble with her schoolwork. She is perfectly attentive in class and does not demonstrate any disruptive or impulsive behaviors. Around her home she helps her mother with chores and is capable of cleaning and dressing herself. She has the most difficulty with reading and according to her mother it takes her "forever" to read a single page of a book. She does poorly on her reading exams and cannot keep up with the rest of her class. At recess she plays well with the other children. What is the approach to the diagnosis of this disorder?

Before making the diagnosis of learning disorder, investigate the potential for poor schooling, language barriers, hearing or vision impairment, communication disorders, mental retardation, and pervasive developmental disorders. In the absence of any functional impairment, this child's specific difficulty with reading as compared to children of her age suggests the diagnosis of learning disorder, or more specifically reading disorder. Five percent of school-age children have learning disorders. They are usually diagnosed by specific intelligence and achievement testing.

A 14-year-old boy recently in trouble for repeated use of profanity in class presents to his primary care physician for evaluation. The boy is sitting in a chair, occasionally grunting and snorting with repetitive eye blinking and throat clearing. He has had terrible difficulty completing his schoolwork lately and admits to using profanity in class. He tells the physician he is aware that shouting profanity in class is wrong but he feels an urge to do so. His father has a similar problem. What is the treatment for this disorder?

Low doses of antipsychotics such as risperidone (Risperdal), ziprasidone (Geodon), haloperidol (Haldol), pimozide (Orap), and fluphenazine (Prolixin) are used to treat Tourette disorder in addition to supportive psychotherapy targeted at minimizing negative social consequences of multiple vocal and motor tics. Tics are sudden, swift, repetitive, arrhythmic, stereotyped movement or vocalization. This boy's coprolalia is an example of a type of vocal tic. Antihypertensive agents (eg, clonidine and guanfacine) are also used to treat tics; studies show variable efficacy, but a lower side effect profile than the antipsychotics.

A 3-year-old boy is brought to his physician by his parents because they have noticed he acts very differently from children of the same age. His parents complain that their son never looks at them in the eye, seems bothered when hugged, never seems to smile, and has not developed much of a vocabulary. In the office, the child faces a corner making a repetitive high-pitched sound while rocking back and forth. When the physician approaches him, the child starts screaming uncontrollably. The child does not respond to his name and is comforted only by a toy car which he shakes incessantly. His parents describe this as his usual behavior in addition to eating according to a very specific time schedule at home. Any alteration in the schedule causes unrest in the child. What disease processes frequently accompany this disorder?

Comorbid seizures and mental retardation frequently accompany autistic disorder; impaired social interactions, impaired communication skills, and a highly limited set of activities and interests characterize autistic disorder. As noted in this child, poor eye contact, lack of facial expression, and poor response to social cues are among the most frequent initial disturbances noted in patients with autistic disorder. Behaviors and interests are described as restrictive, repetitive, and inflexible. This disorder belongs to the spectrum of pervasive developmental disorders. Twenty-five percent of children with autistic disorder have comorbid seizures and 75% have mental retardation.

A 14-month-old child presents to her local ER with a seizure. She has never had a seizure before this one. Her parents have not noticed any problems with their daughter since birth. She has had regular checkups with her pediatrician. Until recently she has played with other children, used her hand to hold and drink from a cup, walked, built towers made of blocks, and said "mama" and "dada." Over the last few weeks her parents noticed a big change in her behavior. She no longer called her parents by name, could not feed herself or drink from a cup, and developed repetitive hand movements. What is the diagnosis?

Rett disorder; an initial period of normal development followed by numerous deficits and neurologic decline suggests the diagnosis of Rett disorder. This disorder is seen in females and thought to have a genetic cause. Children with Rett disorder appear to develop normally until 6-18 months of age when they enter a period of regression characterized by deceleration of head growth; loss of hand coordination; onset of unusual; repetitive hand movements; loss of social; engagement; and eventually severe retardation.

A 5-year-old boy is brought to his pediatrician by his mother because she is unable to leave him alone without him getting extremely upset. She does not understand why this keeps happening because her family members are all so close to each other. When it is time for him to go to school and her to work, the boy suddenly has a terrible bellyache and begins screaming and crying, refusing to go to school. What is the diagnosis of this disorder?

Separation anxiety disorder; refusal to go to school or to sleep alone, somatic symptoms such as stomach or headache, and crying or screaming when being physically separated are all symptoms of separation anxiety disorder. After 3 years of age these behaviors are considered pathologic and may on occasion progress to panic attacks. Children with this disorder fear that harm will come to themselves or to their loved ones on separation. Separation anxiety disorder is most effectively treated with behavioral psychotherapy.

A 9-year-old boy is brought to his family physician by his mother because he has been getting in trouble at school and doing poorly in his classes. He calls out answers in class without being called on. His teacher describes him as very "fidgety." He is caught staring out the window several times a day and requires his teacher's direction to remember what he was doing. He treats his fellow classmates well without any violent or larcenous behavior. His mother comments that at home he starts projects around the house and never finishes them. When he sits down to do his homework he is frequently distracted by almost anything in his environment. This behavior has persisted for 2 years. What is the treatment and dosage strategy for this disorder?

Treat attention deficit hyperactivity disorder (ADHD) with methylphenidate (Ritalin) or dextroamphetamine (Adderall) prescribed at the lowest effective dose; hyperactivity, poor impulse control, inattention, distractibility, and disruptiveness in class are behaviors frequently seen in children with ADHD. The diagnosis requires the onset of inattentive, hyperactive, or impulsive symptoms before age 7. The symptoms must be present in two or more settings with a duration exceeding 6 months. All preparations of methylphenidate and dextroamphetamine (short- and intermediate-acting, and extended release) are equally effective for the treatment of ADHD. Pharmacologic treatment enables improvements in academic performance and avoidance of behavioral complications of the disorder. Nonpharmacologic treatments for ADHD include behavioral strategies such as positive reinforcement for appropriate behaviors and task completion, limit setting, and tailoring environmental stimulation to manageable levels.

CHAPTER 7

Cognitive Disorders

What are the cognitive disorders?

Delirium, dementia, and amnestic disorders

DELIRIUM

! **What is delirium?**

An acute, **fluctuating**, and **transient** disturbance of consciousness accompanied by confusion or other changes in cognition

Epidemiology and Etiology

Are there any gender disparities in the incidence of delirium?

No. Males and females are affected equally.

What percentage of the general medical population develops delirium?

10%-25% of patients over the age of 65. Delirium occurs more frequently in children and in the elderly.

In what two settings is delirium most frequently seen?

Postoperatively and in the intensive care unit

! **What are the common causes of delirium?**

Most commonly the cause is multifactorial, but often may be a result of a general medical condition or substance abuse.

STUPID In THe PM

Seizure (post-ictal from a generalized seizure or non-convulsive status epilepticus)

Toxins (carbon monoxide, organophosphates)

Uremia

Pills (anticholinergics, antibiotics, meperidine, anesthetics)

Infections (urinary tract infections, meningitis, sepsis)

Drug withdrawal (alcohol, benzodiazepines, barbiturates)

Intoxication (alcohol, hallucinogens, opioids, marijuana, stimulants, sedatives)

Thyroid (hyper or hypo)

Head trauma

Postoperative

Metabolic (hyponatremia, hepatic encephalopathy hypoxia, hypercarbia, hypoglycemia, hypo-/hypervolemia, hypercalcemia)

Diagnosis

! **What are the *DSM-IV* (*Diagnostic and Statistical Manual of Mental Disorders, Fourth Edition*) criteria for the diagnosis of delirium?**

1. Changes in attention or arousal
2. Changes in cognition
3. Changes come on acutely and fluctuate throughout the course of the day

! **What is the time course of the development of delirium?**

Acute (hours) or subacute (days). Not chronic!

What is an essential part of the history in a patient suspected to have delirium?

Exhaustive search for any existing medical conditions or substances (illicit as well as prescribed) that could be precipitants of acute mental status change

How may a state of delirium manifest throughout the course of a day?

"Waxing and waning." The patient may have periods of complete clarity mixed with confusion. Sleep-wake cycles may be disturbed. Symptoms may also become worse at night with increased agitation and confusion.

What are the most important parts of the physical examination in the evaluation for delirium?

- Assess mental status using questions about orientation or the mini-mental examination
- Take vital signs with respect to presence or absence of fever, tachycardia, or decreased oxygen saturation
- Observe the patient's general appearance looking for psychomotor agitation or hallucinatory behavior
- Examine the pupils, assess fluid status, and look for signs of infection or underlying systemic diseases

! **Which laboratory or imaging tests are useful in the diagnosis of delirium?**

Finger stick for blood glucose, urinalysis, urine culture, urine toxicology screen, blood culture, complete blood count, electrolytes, blood urea nitrogen (BUN), creatinine, arterial blood gas. In some patients, chest x-ray, head computed tomography (CT), lumbar puncture (LP), electroencephalography (EEG), or magnetic resonance imaging (MRI) may also be useful.

! **What finding on electroencephalography (EEG) is characteristic of delirium?**

Nonspecific, diffuse generalized slowing in the delta and theta range

! **What is the 1-year mortality rate associated with the presence of delirium?**

35%-40%

What does the differential diagnosis of delirium include?

Dementia, psychotic disorder, mania, complex partial seizure

Can delirium exist at the same time as dementia?

Yes, but it is difficult to diagnose a dementia in the presence of delirium.

Treatment

! **What is the primary goal in the initial treatment of delirium?**

Identify and treat any life-threatening conditions that may be presenting with delirium. Also keep patients safe from harming themselves or falling (ie, by using guard rails or bed alarms).

What efforts with regards to a patient's environment can be made to treat and prevent delirium?

Make every attempt to reorient the patient to person, time, and place using verbal cues as well as visual reminders such as easy-to-read calendars and clocks in an appropriately lit room.

! **What is the main treatment of delirium?**

Identify and correct the underlying medical or substance-related condition. This may involve removing offending anticholinergic (or other) medications in the elderly, volume resuscitation, electrolyte correction, using a benzodiazepine to treat alcohol withdrawal, treating infections appropriately, and/or correcting acid/base disorders.

What are the pharmacologic treatments available to treat agitation in delirium?

Low-dose antipsychotics may be used, but caution must be exercised, as these medications are associated with increased mortality in elderly patients with dementia.

! **What psychiatric medications should be avoided?**

SSRIs and benzodiazepines can worsen delirium.

DEMENTIA

What is dementia?

A general loss of cognitive abilities, including impairment of memory as well as one or more of the following: aphasia, apraxia, agnosia, or impaired executive functioning. These cognitive changes are progressive and chronic and are likely due to damage of the central nervous system (CNS).

What is aphasia?

A disorder of speech involving loss of expression, writing, or comprehension of spoken or written language. For example, a patient is unable to name an object held in front of him or her or unable to describe a picture.

What is apraxia?	Loss of ability to carry out familiar, purposeful movements in the absence of paralysis or other motor or sensory impairment. For example, a patient is unable to comb his or her hair or make a cup of tea even though he or she can move his or her extremities without any difficulty or impairment.
What is agnosia?	Loss of the power to recognize sensory stimuli: auditory, gustatory, olfactory, tactile, or visual. For example, a patient is unable to recognize familiar faces (ie, prosopagnosia).
What is impaired executive functioning?	Disturbed planning, organizing, or abstract thinking abilities. For example, a patient is unable to recall the steps necessary to pay a bill with a check, place correct postage on the envelope, and send it in the mail.

Epidemiology and Etiology

Are there any gender disparities in the incidence of dementia?	No. Males and females are affected equally.
How does the prevalence of dementia change with age?	Prevalence increases with age: 2%-5% over age 65 and up to 20% over age 85.
What are some risk factors for developing dementia?	Factors differ according to specific type of dementia but in general include genetic predispositions, cerebrovascular and cardiovascular disease, head trauma, increasing age, and infectious processes.
What is the ultimate pathologic process responsible for dementia, regardless of specific etiology?	Cortical or subcortical neuron loss
! **What is the most common cause of dementia?**	Alzheimer disease accounts for greater than 50% of all dementia.
! **How does the prevalence of Alzheimer disease change with age?**	It doubles every 5 years after age 65. Nearly half of all people age 85 and older have symptoms of Alzheimer disease.
What are the risk factors for Alzheimer disease?	Familial, **Down syndrome**, past head trauma, **increasing age**

What is the link between Alzheimer disease and Down syndrome?	Chromosome 21: trisomy 21 and amyloid precursor protein (APP) on chromosome 21
What is the cleavage product of APP on chromosome 21?	Aβ amyloid results from the breakdown of the protein coded for by the APP gene and is deposited in neuritic plaques leading to excess cerebral amyloid.
Describe the course of Alzheimer disease.	Progressive, with death occurring about 10 years after onset
What is Lewy body dementia?	Disease marked by fluctuating cognition (with great variations in attention and alertness over hours/days), motor features of parkinsonism, and recurrent visual hallucinations
! **What is the second most common cause of dementia?**	Vascular (used to be called "multi-infarct")
! **Name the risk factors associated with vascular dementia.**	Cerebrovascular or cardiovascular disease, hypertension
Describe the course of vascular dementia.	May be acutely or slowly progressive. Further progression may be prevented by appropriate treatment of underlying cerebrovascular or cardiovascular disease as the extent of dementia is determined by cumulative effects of multiple cortical and subcortical infarcts. **Classically demonstrates a stepwise deterioration.**
! **What are the typical presenting symptoms of vascular dementia?**	Presenting symptoms of vascular dementia tend to be more variable than those of Alzheimer disease and can include deficits in executive function, language, and behavior in addition to memory, as well as focal signs corresponding to CNS lesions.
What infectious process may be responsible for dementia in a patient with certain sexual or intravenous drug use risk factors?	Human immunodeficiency virus (HIV) that directly attacks neurons in the white matter or cortex. Acquired immunodeficiency syndrome (AIDS) associated illnesses such as toxoplasmosis or lymphoma may result in dementia; however, they are considered dementia secondary to a general medical condition.

! **What type of dementia is most common in young males?**	Dementia secondary to head trauma
What is the course of dementia resulting from head trauma?	Dementia resulting from head trauma is determined by the extent of the injury. This form of dementia is not progressive unless further head trauma occurs.
What percentage of patients with Parkinson disease develops dementia?	20%-60%
! **What is the proposed etiology of Parkinson disease?**	Progressive loss of dopaminergic neurons in the substantia nigra of the midbrain
What protein is implicated in the development of Parkinson disease and Lewy body dementia?	Alpha-synuclein
What form of dementia is associated with autosomal dominant inheritance on chromosome 4?	Huntington dementia
! **When is the typical age of onset of Huntington dementia?**	In the middle of the third decade of life. However, this disease shows "**anticipation**," which means that the symptoms become apparent at earlier ages in subsequent generations.
When is the typical age of onset of Pick dementia?	Age 50-60
What form of dementia may be attributed to familial or infectious etiology?	Creutzfeldt-Jakob; 10% are considered familial.
What is the agent of transmission in Creutzfeldt-Jakob?	An infectious protein called a prion
What is the typical age of onset of Creutzfeldt-Jakob?	Onset usually occurs between 40 and 60 years of age.
! **Describe the typical course of Creutzfeldt-Jakob.**	Rapidly progressive and fatal within 1 year
What are examples of dementia due to metabolic disorders?	Diseases of myelin; Wilson disease (excess copper); diseases of carbohydrate, lipid, and protein metabolism; uremic encephalopathy

! What is an endocrinologic cause of dementia?

Hypothyroidism (Remember to measure thyroid-stimulating hormone [TSH]!)

What is an example of a steroid responsive encephalopathy that could present as a rapidly progressive dementia?

Hashimoto encephalopathy

What type of dementia can be associated with amyotrophic lateral sclerosis (ALS)?

Fronto-temporal dementia

What types of exogenous substances may result in dementias?

Alcohol, anticonvulsants, chemotherapeutics, inhalants, sedatives, heavy metals, solvents, pesticides

! What are examples of reversible or partially reversible dementias?

Normal pressure hydrocephalus (NPH), neurosyphilis, thiamine, folate, vitamin B_{12}, and niacin deficiencies

Diagnosis

! What are the *DSM-IV* criteria for diagnosis of dementia?

- Memory loss
- Loss of one or more cognitive abilities including aphasia, apraxia, agnosia, or impaired executive functioning:
  - These disturbances must exist after any state of superimposed delirium has resolved.
  - These disturbances must impair social or occupational functioning.
  - These disturbances must represent a decline from previous level of functioning.

! How does the onset of dementia differ from that of delirium?

Delirium develops acutely or subacutely within hours to days. Dementia has more of a chronic onset of weeks to years.

! How does the course of dementia differ from that of delirium?

Delirium fluctuates within a day and may last hours to weeks with resolution. Dementia behaves in a more stable fashion with deficits that can be permanent, reversible, or progressive over weeks to years.

What does the term "sundowning" refer to?

The worsening of cognitive symptoms including memory deficits, agitation, and disturbances in attention at night. This may be characteristic of delirium as well as dementia.

What is the approach to the diagnosis of dementia?

- History of memory and cognitive impairment
- Mental status examination, especially the "**Mini-mental state examination (MMSE)**"
  - General medical examination with attention to signs of atherosclerosis (carotid bruits, abdominal aortic aneurysm [AAA]) and chronic encephalopathic states (liver disease, uremia)
- Complete neurologic examination
  - Lab studies of electrolytes, vitamins (especially folate and B_{12}), toxins, infectious studies (Venereal Disease Research Laboratory [VDRL], fluorescent treponemal antibody [FTA] for syphilis or HIV testing)
- Note that EEG is **not** sensitive for dementia

What findings on mental status examination are characteristic of dementia?

- Memory impairment (especially short-term)
- Impaired recall of names
  - Inability to recognize or name familiar objects
  - Inability to describe sequential or multistep tasks as involved in executive functioning, planning, and organization
- Paranoia
- Hallucinations
- Delusions

What findings are characteristic of late stage dementia?

- Incontinence
- Abulia or complete mutism
- Inability to perform even simple activities of daily living
- Frontal release signs (suck, snout, palmo-mental, grasp)

What is abulia?

Reduction in thought, speech, movement, and emotional reaction

! What is the Mini-mental State Examination (MMSE)?

A brief 30-point questionnaire test that is used to screen for cognitive impairment

! How is the MMSE scored?

>24 points is considered normal. Below this, scores can indicate mild (21-23 points), moderate (10-20 points), or severe (≤9 points) dementia.

What are the gross and microscopic pathologic findings in Alzheimer disease?

- Cortical atrophy
- Loss of forebrain cholinergic nuclei
- **Neurofibrillary tangles**
- **Amyloid plaques composed of abnormal tau proteins**
- Granulovacuolar degeneration

! Describe the clinical findings in Alzheimer disease.

Memory impairment is prominent. Emotional disturbances occur early. There are only minimal focal findings on examination.

! What is mild cognitive impairment (MCI)?

Cognitive impairment beyond that expected for a patient's age/education that does **not** significantly impair functioning. Studies suggest that individuals with MCI progress to Alzheimer disease at a rate of approximately 10%-15% per year.

What findings are characteristic of vascular dementia?

Motor deficits often accompanied by focal CNS lesions and atrophy on neuroimaging

! What are the typical MRI findings in vascular dementia?

Multiple lacunar white matter infarcts

What pathologic findings are associated with Lewy body dementia?

- Lewy body inclusions affecting cortical neurons diffusely
- Absence or inconspicuous number of neurofibrillary tangles and senile plaques

What histologic stains aid in the pathologic diagnosis of Lewy body dementia?

Immunostaining for ubiquitin and synuclein

! What is the nature of the psychosis seen in Lewy body dementia?

Visual hallucinations occur in 75% of people with Lewy body dementia and involve the perception of people or animals that aren't there. These hallucinations are not necessarily disturbing.

What clinical feature may be associated with Parkinson dementia?	Bradyphrenia (slowed thinking)
What is the distinction between Lewy body dementia and Parkinson dementia?	Lewy body dementia is diagnosed when cognitive symptoms begin at the same time or within a year of Parkinsonian symptoms. Parkinson dementia is diagnosed when dementia onset is more than 1 year after the onset of parkinsonism.
What clinical finding is characteristic of Huntington disease?	Choreoathetosis, which is the presence of irregular spasmodic, involuntary movements of the limbs or facial muscles as well as slow, writhing, dance-like involuntary movement of the fingers and hands
What clinical feature is associated with Huntington dementia?	Emotional lability and depression
! **What pathologic finding is associated with Huntington dementia?**	Atrophy of the caudate
! **What neuroimaging finding is suggestive of Huntington disease?**	"Boxcar" ventricles
How does dementia of Pick disease (or frontal-temporal dementia) typically present?	Initially with changes in personality and language in the fifth decade
What is the characteristic neuroimaging finding in Pick dementia?	Frontal and temporal atrophy
! **What is the clinical triad suggestive of Creutzfeldt-Jakob?**	1. Dementia 2. Myoclonus, often with a startle component 3. Abnormal EEG—high-voltage synchronous **sharp waves**
What are the gross and microscopic pathologic findings in Creutzfeldt-Jakob?	Spongiform changes
What is the triad of NPH?	1. "*Wet*"—urinary incontinence 2. "*Wacky*"—dementia and personality changes such as being withdrawn and apathetic 3. "*Wobbly*"—gait abnormality

Which symptom of NPH is generally the first to appear?

In many cases of NPH, the presenting symptom is gait disturbance.

Which symptom of NPH is generally the last to appear?

Incontinence usually occurs in more advanced cases.

How is the dementia of NPH characterized?

Impairments in attention, visuospatial relations, and judgment

How is the diagnosis of NPH confirmed?

- *Lumbar puncture:* normal cerebrospinal fluid pressure
- *Imaging:* dilated ventricles in the absence of cortical atrophy

What does the differential diagnosis of dementia include?

Delirium, developmental disorders with impaired cognition, mental retardation, psychotic disorder, major depression (aka pseudodementia), age-related cognitive decline

How can the pseudodementia of depression be differentiated from dementia?

Specific neuropsychological tests designed to assess intellect, language, learning and memory, attention and concentration, visuospatial skills, mood and personality, motor and sensory skills, and higher executive functioning. Examples include the Luria-Nebraska and Halstead-Reitan test batteries.

How can the mental status examination be used to differentiate pseudodementia from dementia?

	Pseudodementia	Dementia
Mood symptoms	Prominent	Variable
Memory impairment	Reports marked impairment	May be unaware
Response to questioning	Often dismissive; "I don't know"	Nonsense or sometimes elaborate explanations without an answer
Memory testing	Intact with rehearsal	Not intact but often attempts to remember

Treatment

What are the treatment goals for dementia?

- Treat the underlying cause if one exists.
- Provide rehabilitation to manage deficits.
- Consider modified living situations or housing options to ensure optimal patient safety.
- Use pharmacologic therapies to treat symptoms of dementia while avoiding those that further impair cognition.
- Provide reassurance and support to the patient.

What pharmacologic therapy exists to slow the progression of memory loss in Alzheimer dementia?

- Acetylcholinesterase inhibitors: donepezil (Aricept), tacrine (Cognex), rivastigmine (Exelon), galantamine (Razadyne)
- NMDA (*N*-methyl-d-aspartate) receptor antagonists such as memantine (Namenda)

! What pharmacologic therapy exists to treat the agitation, paranoia, and hallucinations of dementia?

Low doses of high-potency antipsychotics. Remember that these medications are associated with a small chance of increased mortality among elderly patients with dementia, so benefits and risks must be carefully weighed.

! In what form of dementia are antipsychotics relatively contraindicated?

Lewy body dementia—antipsychotics may worsen the symptoms of this disease.

Which antipsychotic is recommended for treating psychosis associated with Parkinson dementia?

Clozapine (Clozaril)

How is the dementia of NPH treated?

Cerebrospinal fluid shunt

AMNESTIC DISORDERS

What are amnestic disorders?

Solitary disturbances in memory without any change in alertness or other neurologic or cognitive functions. General medical conditions, substance abuse, or trauma may be responsible for these disturbances.

Epidemiology and Etiology

What risk factors exist for the development of amnestic disorders?	Alcohol and substance abuse, general medical conditions
Name the general medical conditions that can be responsible for amnestic disorders.	Head trauma, hypoxia, herpes simplex encephalitis, posterior cerebral artery infarction
! What is the leading cause of substance-related amnestic disorder?	Alcohol abuse—"blackouts"
Damage to what three brain structures most commonly causes amnestic symptoms?	1. Fornix 2. Hippocampus 3. Mamillary bodies
Which of these brain structures is most susceptible to hypoxic damage?	Hippocampus
Which of these brain structures is characteristically damaged in Wernicke-Korsakoff syndrome?	Mamillary bodies
What is transient global amnesia?	Sudden loss of memory and recent events accompanied by the inability to recall new information or form new memories
When does transient global amnesia typically present?	Middle or elderly age
! Describe the course of transient global amnesia.	Minutes to hours with episodic attacks usually remitting within 24 hours without any residual memory loss upon resolution
How does a patient usually present with transient global amnesia?	Patients are aware of their deficits, often repetitively inquiring about the details of their surroundings or recent events. Consciousness and personal identity are not disturbed. High-level intellectual functioning and language function are intact during the episode.

Diagnosis

What mental status examination features are characteristic of amnestic disorders?	Memory deficits in either previously learned or newly acquired information

Besides memory deficits what other factor must exist for the diagnosis of amnestic disorder?

An identifiable precipitant

What does the differential diagnosis of amnestic disorders include?

Delirium, dementia, alcohol abuse

How can amnestic disorders be differentiated from delirium or dementia?

The presence of cognitive deficits or disturbances in the level of alertness in addition to memory impairment implies that delirium or dementia may be a more accurate diagnosis.

Treatment

What are the primary treatment goals in amnestic disorders?

- Correct underlying medical conditions.
- Treat any existing substance abuse and dependency and avoid further use.
- Ensure a safe environment for the patient with appropriate structure and memory cues.

CLINICAL VIGNETTES

A 59-year-old African American man with a history of hypertension and diabetes is brought to his physician by his son because of "strange behavior." The son notes that his father has had trouble remembering various appointments around town. Recently, his father has needed assistance to find his own way to the Senior Citizen Center, because he can no longer find his way by himself. Apparently, other people at the center have also remarked that the man has not been himself. He has been loud, unusually mean, and has "lost his sense of humor." At home his son has found him talking to an empty room as if there was someone there. On examination, he is uncooperative and demonstrates mild difficulty with memory tasks, but no other neurologic findings. An MRI shows frontal and temporal atrophy. What is the diagnosis?

Pick dementia; the characteristics of memory loss in addition to loss of one or more cognitive abilities with chronic onset support the diagnosis of dementia. Frontal and temporal atrophy are characteristic neuroimaging findings in Pick dementia. This form of dementia usually presents between the ages of 50 and 60 with changes in personality and language being the prominent features of this disease.

A 42-year-old Hispanic woman with a history of mental retardation is brought to her primary care physician by her parents because of "forgetfulness." She has been working at a nearby grocery store bagging groceries for customers over the last 15 years. Her boss called her parents to tell them that she is no longer able to function at her job. She appears as if she does not know what to do with the groceries. She has been showing up late and even got lost on her usual walk to the store from her house. At work she has uncharacteristically been making sexual advances on some of the customers. When her parents ask her about her day at work she has difficulty remembering what happened. On examination, she has a flat face with a short nose, prominent epicanthic skin folds, small low-set ears, a thick tongue, and a single transverse palmar crease. She has difficulty with short-term memory, calculation, and sequential tasks. What is the etiologic link between the two diagnoses this patient carries?

The amyloid precursor protein (APP) gene on chromosome 21 is the etiologic link between Down syndrome and Alzheimer disease; with the history of mental retardation and characteristic physical findings it is clear that this patient has Down syndrome. The most common cause of Down syndrome is trisomy 21. Almost all patients over 30 years of age with Down syndrome develop the plaques and neurofibrillary tangles characteristic of Alzheimer disease. The gene APP has been implicated in some cases of early onset, autosomal dominant Alzheimer disease. The APP gene is located on chromosome 21. Aβ amyloid results from the breakdown of the protein coded for by the APP gene and is deposited in neuritic plaques. Considering these genetic findings, it has been proposed that an extra copy of the APP gene from a trisomy of chromosome 21 leads to excess cerebral amyloid and thus the Alzheimer dementia seen in Down syndrome patients.

An 86-year-old man with a history of hypertension, diabetes, and chronic obstructive pulmonary disease (COPD) is hospitalized for congestive heart failure. He has been in the hospital for 4 days and has been receiving furosemide and metoprolol in addition to his regular medications, which include hydrochlorothiazide, lisinopril, Protonix, metformin, insulin, albuterol inhaler, ipratropium bromide inhaler, and aspirin. He has had a Foley catheter for 3 days because he has been too weak to get out of bed to use the bathroom. According to his family, he is a very mild mannered, pleasant gentleman at home; however, over the last hour the nurses have complained that he has been yelling at them, trying to get out of bed, and talking to people who are not actually in the room. At times he appears calm and sleepy, and then he shifts back into the behavior described by the nurses. Over the last few hours he has also developed a cough. What is the approach to diagnosis and treatment in this patient?

Delirium; identify and treat any life-threatening conditions then search for other underlying causes; this patient is an elderly man with a significant medical history on a prolonged hospital stay. His waxing and waning course of confusion and agitation suggests delirium over dementia. Yelling, restlessness, changes in consciousness, and hallucinations are all manifestations of delirium. Whenever a patient presents with delirium, an extensive search for the underlying cause must be undertaken. Elderly age is a risk factor for the development of delirium. He is taking multiple medications including ipratropium, the anticholinergic properties of which can cause delirium. An elderly person who has stayed in the hospital for a few days is at risk for infection, another frequent cause of delirium. Sources of infection for this patient include nosocomial pneumonia, as suggested by the acute onset of cough, and urinary tract infection, as suggested by having a bladder catheter in place for more than 3 days. Vital signs, physical examination, electrolytes, white blood count, chest x-ray, urinalysis, and urine and blood cultures are appropriate for this patient. If the urinalysis is positive for infection, his urinary catheter should be removed. In this patient's case it may be necessary to insert a new, sterile catheter to achieve diuresis in the setting of congestive heart failure. Depending on the results of these steps, empiric antibiotics may be warranted until cultures allow the antimicrobial spectrum to be narrowed. This patient's medications should also be reviewed, and any extraneous agents should be eliminated. Health care providers should make every attempt to ensure the patient's safety, reorient him to the environment, and evaluate the appropriateness of using low-dose antipsychotic medication if agitation becomes marked.

A 52-year-old woman is brought to the hospital by a local policeman because she presented to the police station asking about where she was. She does not recognize any parts of the city around her. She is able to correctly identify herself and remains alert without any trouble speaking or slurring of speech. She denies alcohol or drug use. The physical examination is completely normal except for memory testing. The last thing she remembers is being with her husband and two children 3 hours ago but has no idea where they are or where she is now. After 2 hours of observation in the hospital while the physicians attempt to locate her family, she suddenly remembers exactly where she is and has no further memory deficit. What is the diagnosis?

Transient global amnesia; sudden loss of memory and recent events accompanied by the inability to recall new information suggests the diagnosis of transient global amnesia. This disorder typically presents in middle or elderly age. Attacks are episodic, lasting between minutes to hours and usually resolving within 24 hours without any residual memory loss. Note that this woman was aware of her deficits and retained her personal identity. She inquired mostly about the details of her surroundings. There was no impairment of executive functioning or language.

A 37-year-old homeless man is brought into the ED after being picked up by the emergency medical technicians (EMTs) in front of an outdoor café. Apparently the man was yelling at the customers seated at tables about nonsensical things. He kept asking them why he was at the zoo. On examination, he was disheveled, malodorous, and confused. He had trouble keeping his balance and walking a straight line. On extraocular muscle examination, the physician asked him to follow a finger out to his right side with his eyes while keeping his head straight ahead. His left eye moved medially to his nose while his right eye could not move laterally to the finger. BAL was elevated. What is the treatment for this disease process?

Wernicke encephalopathy, treat with immediate intravenous thiamine infusion; prolonged alcohol abuse leads to thiamine deficiency. Because the mamillary bodies and dorsomedial nucleus of the thalamus are dependent on thiamine, its deficiency may result in Wernicke-Korsakoff syndrome. This patient demonstrates the classical triad of ataxia, abnormal eye movements including nystagmus and lateral gaze palsy, and confusion.

A 39-year-old white man with a history of hypertension presents to his primary care physician with his wife because of "forgetfulness." People around him have commented that he seems to forget conversations, appointments, and recent events. His wife has also noticed strange movements of his upper extremities, which she describes as "dance-like." He has been dropping things lately, such as his morning cup of coffee that "just doesn't seem to stay in his hand." On examination, the man is calm and pleasant with slightly elevated blood pressure. Occasionally, there are slow, writhing movements of his hands, arm, and neck. Examination of the eye reveals golden brown pigmentation on the posterior corneal surface. Lab work shows normal CBC and electrolyte panel. A test for serum ceruloplasmin is low. What is the diagnosis?

Wilson disease; Wilson disease is characterized by excess copper due to a deficiency of the copper-carrying protein ceruloplasmin, which can be measured in the serum as it was in this patient. Also termed hepatolenticular degeneration, Wilson disease is an autosomal recessive disorder which presents most often between 20 and 40 years of age. Psychiatric disturbances in this disorder include changes in personality and mood disturbances. Neurologic symptoms may include impairments in memory and executive functioning, difficulty with coordination, gait disturbances, choreiform movements, tremor, and rigidity. The golden brown pigmentation of this patient's posterior corneal surface, or Kayser-Fleischer ring, is a characteristic finding of this disease.

A 72-year-old woman with a history of congestive heart failure presents to the ED with shortness of breath. She is admitted to a general medical team and over the course of 2 days she receives furosemide for diuresis, and her cardiac markers are assessed to rule out a myocardial infarction. She remains in her hospital bed throughout much of her hospital course. During the middle of the third night she is found by the nurse to be climbing out of bed and calling out her deceased husband's name. The patient becomes agitated as the nurse attempts to reassure her. Eventually the nurse coaxes her to return to bed. Soon after this incident as morning begins, the patient becomes difficult to arouse. On examination, the patient's temperature is 101°F, BP 134/84 mm Hg, HR 95. As she is examined the patient becomes agitated again. She is coughing and rhonchi are heard in the right middle lung field as well as bibasilar crackles. Cardiac examination is unchanged. Abdominal examination is benign. Extremity examination reveals pitting edema improving from previous examinations. How can this patient's cognitive state best be described? What is the likely underlying diagnosis?

Delirium most likely secondary to hospital-acquired pneumonia; this patient's acute, fluctuating, and transient disturbance of consciousness accompanied by confusion and other changes in cognition is indicative of delirium. It is important to recognize that delirium is not a diagnosis but rather a sign that there exists some underlying, potentially life-threatening medical condition. Simply staying in a hospital for a few days is a risk factor for an elderly person to develop a hospital-acquired pneumonia. The fact that the patient is febrile, coughing, and has findings on pulmonary auscultation supports a diagnosis of pneumonia. Further tests such as white blood cell count, sputum culture, chest x-ray, and electrolytes are warranted to make the diagnosis as well as rule out other causes of delirium. Empiric treatment of the suspected pneumonia with antibiotics should be initiated until an organism is identified or some other diagnosis becomes more appropriate with further workup.

An 82-year-old white woman with a history of hypertension and diabetes is brought to her physician by her daughter because of "forgetfulness." At first, the daughter noticed only that her mother would not remember phone conversations with her. Recently, she has visited her mother's house to find the stove left on, clothes scattered about the house, and an answering machine full of messages regarding missed lunch appointments with friends. A week ago, a neighbor brought her mother back home after finding her lost in the town's center. On examination, she demonstrates difficulty with word finding, immediate recall, recent memory, and sequential tasks. The patient answers questions accurately about her childhood and does not seem to think that there is anything wrong with her. What are the gross and microscopic pathologic findings in patients with this disease?

Alzheimer disease: cortical atrophy, neurofibrillary tangles, and amyloid plaques; the characteristics of memory loss in addition to loss of one or more cognitive abilities (in this case aphasia and impaired executive functioning) with chronic onset support the diagnosis of dementia. Alzheimer disease is ultimately a pathologic diagnosis; however, prominent memory loss with minimal focal findings on examination makes this the appropriate classification of dementia in this case. Gross pathologic findings include cortical atrophy. Microscopic pathologic findings include loss of forebrain cholinergic nuclei, neurofibrillary tangles, amyloid plaques composed of abnormal tau proteins, and granulovacuolar degeneration. Pharmacologic therapy to treat memory loss in Alzheimer dementia includes acetylcholinesterase inhibitors and *N*-methyl-D-aspartic acid (NMDA) receptor antagonists.

An 84-year-old white woman with a history of hypertension is admitted to the hospital for dehydration and malnutrition. Four months ago, her son brought her to their family physician because of "forgetfulness." At first the son noticed only that his mother would not remember conversations she had with him. Recently, he visited his mother's house to find the stove left on, odd piles of random objects scattered about the house, overflowing trash cans, and an answering machine full of messages regarding missed appointments with friends. An examination at that time demonstrated difficulty with word finding, immediate recall, recent memory, and sequential tasks. The patient answered questions accurately about her childhood and did not seem to think that there was anything wrong with her. During this hospitalization she is highly agitated and refuses to eat. In contrast to her behavior over the last 4 months, the patient has periods of complete clarity mixed with confusion that is worse at night. Her sleep-wake cycles are also disturbed. Her physical examination is notable for orthostatic hypotension, dry mucous membranes, and decreased skin turgor. How can this woman's mental status be best described? What is the most likely underlying cause?

Delirium most likely secondary to dehydration in an Alzheimer patient; this woman has dementia most likely of the Alzheimer type, as suggested by characteristics of memory loss in addition to loss of one or more cognitive abilities such as aphasia and impaired executive functioning. It is important to note that delirium can be superimposed on an existing dementia. As the 1-year mortality of delirium approaches 35%-40%, detecting delirium in a patient with dementia can be lifesaving. This patient was admitted with dehydration and the physical findings of orthostatic hypotension, dry mucous membranes, and decreased skin turgor suggest that she remains volume depleted. Volume depletion can cause acute changes in attention, arousal, and cognition characteristic of delirium. Careful volume repletion, as well as correcting any electrolyte abnormality, is necessary in this case. The patient should also be kept safe from harming herself or falling. Despite the underlying dementia, every attempt should be made to reorient the patient to person, time, and place using verbal cues as well as visual reminders such as easy-to-read calendars and clocks in an appropriately lit room.

A 35-year-old white man with a history of hypertension and diabetes is brought to his family physician by his wife because she noticed he has been feeling "down" lately. He has started to have sudden irregular movements of his face and extremities. These movements have been uncontrollable and remind him of his father who had similar problems before dying. His wife describes a sense of worthlessness, a change in sleeping pattern, and an extreme moodiness in her husband. Recently, she has noticed him swatting his hands in the air and calling out as if he was speaking to someone. What is the specific inheritance pattern of the disease underlying this state of dementia?

Huntington disease exhibits autosomal dominant inheritance and is associated with trinucleotide repeat expansion on chromosome 4p; Huntington disease is an autosomal dominant disorder with complete penetrance. The mutation is due to a trinucleotide (CAG) repeat expansion in the Huntington gene on chromosome 4p. The typical onset is in the middle of the third decade of life. The sudden irregular movements of this patient's face and extremities are termed choreoathetosis, which may also present as slow, writhing, dance-like involuntary flexion, extension, pronation, and supination of the fingers and hands. The underlying pathology of this disturbance in movement is atrophy of the caudate. This patient's depressed mood is characteristic of the emotional lability associated with Huntington dementia.

A 54-year-old man is brought to the hospital by the police after causing trouble at home. The man works as a wood carver. He was in the Navy for 25 years until he was dishonorably discharged because of continued alcohol abuse. Over the last 4 years, he has been living with his elderly parents who refuse to deal with his alcohol problem any longer. The parents report that their son cannot hold a job, rarely sells a piece of his wood carving, and makes a mess at home. When questioning the man, he is slightly confused and perseverates about his skill as a wood carver. He is able to recount the earlier years of his Navy career, but is unable to account for the happenings of the last 7 years. He cannot exactly remember when or why he left the Navy. On memory testing, he is able to repeat three words immediately after the physician says them; however, he can remember only one of the words after 3 minutes and none of the words after 5 minutes. He is unaware of current political, local, or world events. What is the most likely diagnosis?

Korsakoff syndrome; alcohol abuse is a leading cause of substance-related amnestic disorder. Korsakoff syndrome (alcohol-induced persistent amnestic disorder) can persist after proper treatment of Wernicke encephalopathy with thiamine infusion. The diagnosis of Korsakoff syndrome is appropriate in this patient because of his long-standing alcohol abuse history, impaired short-term memory, and permanent gap in memory of a definitive period in time due to anterograde amnesia. Persons with Korsakoff syndrome are known to confabulate to compensate for their memory loss. Damage to the mamillary bodies causes the amnestic symptoms seen in Wernicke-Korsakoff syndrome. Two-thirds of Korsakoff cases are irreversible but thiamine and folate should be supplemented.

A 78-year-old white man with a history of hypertension and diabetes is brought to the ER after he was found wandering the town square. He told the EMTs that he knew he had something to do in that area but forgot what it was. When the man's daughter arrived at the hospital she reports that he recently has not been able to recall the events of the last few years. She also remarks that he never liked to take his blood pressure medication. On examination, he is slow in responding to questions and often cannot complete a sentence because he cannot think of a particular word. He demonstrates impairment in short-term memory. Further examination reveals right upper and lower extremity weakness as well as extensor plantar reflexes and a BP of 190/110 mm Hg. How may further progression of this form of dementia be prevented?

Vascular dementia, treat underlying risk factors to avoid progression; this patient's aphasia and memory impairment in the setting of a history of presumably uncontrolled hypertension and neurologic deficits including motor weakness and present Babinski signs suggests multi-infarct or vascular dementia, the second most common cause of dementia. The onset of vascular dementia is sudden and progresses in a stepwise fashion. Presenting symptoms of vascular dementia tend to be more variable than with Alzheimer disease (ie, deficits in executive function, language, and behavior in addition to memory). As hypertension, cerebrovascular, and cardiovascular disease are risk factors for vascular dementia, treatment of these processes may prevent further progression of the dementia. The extent of dementia is determined by cumulative effects of multiple cortical and subcortical infarcts. Neuroimaging may show multiple white matter lacunar infarcts.

A 66-year-old retired army veteran with a history of hypertension and diabetes is admitted to the hospital for pneumonia. He received appropriate antibiotic therapy and was placed on an insulin sliding scale for diabetes. On hospital day number 2, the patient suddenly becomes agitated and starts yelling at the nurses. He seems to be drifting in and out of sleep. On examination, his temperature is 100.5°F, BP 145/95 mm Hg, HR 110, and RR 22. He is noted to be tremulous. The remainder of his examination is unremarkable. What term best describes this man's symptoms? What is the most likely underlying cause?

Delirium most likely secondary to alcohol withdrawal; changes in attention and arousal, or "waxing and waning," over an acute time course suggest that delirium is responsible for this man's change in mental status. The diagnostic workup for delirium includes assessing mental status; obtaining vital signs with respect to presence or absence of fever, tachycardia, or decreased oxygen saturation; observing the patient's general appearance for psychomotor agitation or hallucinatory behavior; examining the pupils, assessing fluid status, and looking for signs of infection or underlying systemic diseases. This patient has an elevated temperature in the setting of tachycardia and tremulousness after being in the hospital for 2 days. An accurate social history at the time of admission may have documented alcohol use but regardless of this information the suspicion for alcohol or benzodiazepine withdrawal should be high. Alcohol withdrawal needs to be treated urgently with benzodiazepines to avoid progression of withdrawal to life-threatening delirium tremens. Many institutions have protocols in place for the routine assessment of withdrawal symptoms and their prompt treatment.

A 79-year-old man is brought to your office by his family, who claim that in the past year he has been having increasing problems with his memory. They say that he often forgets people's names, misplaces items, and gets lost in familiar surroundings. He also has been showing more difficulty with basic tasks such as eating, dressing, and bathing himself. You perform a Mini-mental State Exam and the patient scores a 15. The patient's physical exam is within normal limits. What is the most likely diagnosis, and what treatment should you offer?

The patient has moderate to severe dementia. The most likely diagnosis is Alzheimer disease, which accounts for more than 50% of cases of dementia. Moreover, this patient's clinical presentation is consistent with Alzheimer disease in that he is displaying prominent memory deficits and has no focal physical findings. The most appropriate treatment for this patient would be memantine (Namenda), which is indicated in moderate to severe dementia (ie, MMSE<16) and is known to have a modest effect on the progression of dementia.

CHAPTER 8

Somatoform Disorders, Factitious Disorders, and Malingering

What is somatization?

A tendency to experience and communicate somatic distress in response to psychosocial stress and to seek medical help for it

What key factor allows one to differentiate between various forms of somatization?

Whether this process is employed consciously or unconsciously

! **What is the difference between somatoform disorders and factitious disorders?**

- Somatoform = *unconscious* production of physical signs and symptoms of illness
- Factitious = *conscious* production of complaints to assume "sick role"

What is the difference between factitious disorders and malingering?

- Goal of factitious = primary gain
- Goal of malingering = secondary gain

What is primary gain?

Assuming the *sick role* to obtain the psychological benefit of being cared for and receiving attention from nurturing, authoritative figures

What is secondary gain?

Some benefit arising from being ill that is recognizable to the observer

! **What are examples of secondary gain?**

- Financial benefit in the form of disability pay
- Medications such as pain pills
- Decisions made by health care workers to support pending legal cases
- Avoiding commitments such as military service or work obligations

In what health care setting do most patients with somatization present?

Primary care offices

What effect does somatization have on the health care system?

Increases utilization of care and health care expenditure

When a patient presents with somatization what potential underlying problems should be investigated?

- Underlying psychiatric syndrome
- Coexisting personality disorder
- Psychosocial stressor such as sexual abuse

What elements of history are suggestive of somatoform disorders?

Several unconnected, exaggerated, often strange medical complaints that have been worked up by numerous physicians in the past without clear cause

What elements of examination and laboratory studies are suggestive of somatoform disorders?

Anxiety about these complaints, strange indifference to significant medical complaints, inconsistent physical examination or lab findings

SOMATIZATION DISORDER

Epidemiology and Etiology

What age group has the highest incidence of somatization disorder?

16-25 years of age

! **What gender presents with somatization disorder more frequently?**

20:1 female to male ratio

In what socioeconomic class is somatization disorder more common?

Lower socioeconomic group

Is there a familial pattern with somatization disorder?

Yes, incidence is increased in first-degree relatives.

! **Are physical signs and symptoms consciously produced by the patient?**

No

Male relatives of patients with somatization disorder are more likely to manifest which disorders?

Antisocial personality disorder and substance abuse

What environmental factors are prevalent among patients with somatization disorder?

History of illness in the family or **history of abusive relationships**

Diagnosis

! **When should somatization disorder be suspected?**

Multiple medical complaints (diffusely positive review of systems) without any medical cause

! **What are the *DSM-IV* (*Diagnostic and Statistical Manual of Mental Disorders, Fourth Edition*) criteria for diagnosis of somatization disorder?**

- History of seeking treatment for several physical complaints beginning before age 30 and occurring over several years
- Functional impairment results from these complaints
- Presence of **each** of the following at any time during the course:
  - *Pain symptoms* (four or more) involving multiple sites or systems
  - *Gastrointestinal symptoms* other than pain (two or more)
  - *Sexual symptom* (one or more) other than pain
  - *Pseudoneurologic symptom* (one or more) other than pain
- None of these symptoms are intentionally produced or feigned

What is the temporal relationship between the presenting symptoms and diagnosis?

The symptoms must have begun before the age of 30 and have lasted for several years.

What does the differential diagnosis for somatization disorder include?

Mood and anxiety disorders with physical complaints, schizophrenia with somatic delusions, other somatoform disorders, factitious disorders, malingering, general medical condition, fibromyalgia

Treatment

What goals should guide treatment of somatization disorder?

- Recognition of the disorder so as to avoid further unnecessary workup
- Proper documentation of the disorder to enhance collaboration among other health care providers participating in diagnosis and management
- Involvement of psychiatric services to provide appropriate support and identify comorbid disorders or psychosocial stressors
- Recognition that morbidity may be somewhat alleviated with appropriate support but cure is rarely achieved

! **How should physicians optimally interact with patients affected by somatization disorder?**

Focus on psychological impact of symptoms instead of continuing medical workup or prescribing unnecessary analgesics or anxiolytics

What is the key to successful treatment of somatization disorder?

Formation of a therapeutic doctor-patient relationship with **regular follow-up**

What is the prognosis for somatization disorder?

Poor to fair with manifestations of the disorder recurring throughout one's life

CONVERSION DISORDER

What is conversion disorder?

The presence of one or more motor or sensory symptoms that has a severe impact on activities of daily living or functionality

Epidemiology and Etiology

! **What age group presents with conversion disorder?**

Conversion disorder may present at any age but is rare in children younger than 10 years or in the elderly. Studies suggest a peak onset in the mid-to-late 30s.

! **What gender presents with conversion disorder more frequently?**

5:1 female to male ratio

In what socioeconomic class is conversion disorder more common?

Lower socioeconomic groups with rural background and poor education

What comorbid conditions are associated with conversion disorder?

Drug and alcohol dependence, sociopathic personality, somatization disorder

Is there a familial pattern with conversion disorder?

Yes

! **Are physical signs and symptoms consciously produced by the patient?**

No

! **What are the likely etiologies of the physical symptoms?**

Stress, conflict, prior sexual abuse

What is the physiologic cause of conversion disorder?

There is no known physiologic cause for the impairment in function brought on by conversion disorder.

In what settings do most conversion disorders present?

Ambulatory settings, emergency departments, neurology service

Diagnosis

! **What are the *DSM-IV* criteria for the diagnosis of conversion disorder?**

1. Symptoms: one or more involving voluntary motor or sensory system more than pain that resemble a neurologic or general medical condition
2. Psychological factors: temporal relationship exists between conflict and physical symptoms
3. Unintentional nature of the symptoms
4. Exclusion of general medical conditions, substance-related cause, or culturally sanctioned behavior
5. Functionality is impaired by existence of symptoms
6. Not better explained by pain or sexual dysfunction, another mental disorder, or occurring exclusively during the course of somatization disorder

! **How do motor symptoms in conversion disorder typically present?**

Paralysis of an extremity

! **How do sensory symptoms in conversion disorder typically present?**	Anesthesia (often in a non-anatomical distribution) or visual disturbances such as blindness
! **Describe the onset of conversion disorder.**	Acute and associated with psychological stress
What subtypes of conversion disorder exist?	Classified by type of symptoms: motor, sensory, seizure, or a mixture
! **How do the symptoms of somatization disorder differ from conversion disorder?**	Patients with somatization disorder have **multiple medical complaints** spread over several body systems, whereas conversion disorder patients typically have a single, prominent, pseudoneurologic symptom associated with a psychological stressor.
What features may be associated with conversion disorder?	• Personality disorders such as antisocial, dependent, histrionic, borderline • Mood disorders or lack of appropriate concern • Dissociative disorders • General medical conditions
What is included in the differential diagnosis of conversion disorder?	General medical conditions, neurologic conditions such as multiple sclerosis or an underlying seizure disorder in patients with pseudoseizures, factitious disorders, malingering

Treatment

! **What is the first step in treatment of conversion disorder?**	Rule out general medical cause
What treatment modalities are commonly employed for conversion disorder?	• Use of suggestion with hypnosis • Relaxation techniques • Psychotherapy • **Reassurance that it will improve**
What is the typical duration of symptoms in conversion disorder?	About 2 weeks or less
What is the prognosis for conversion disorder?	Very good with high response rate to most therapeutic options when presented in a way that is suggestive of a cure. This disorder is usually self-limiting, although it can often recur in the future under stress.

PAIN DISORDER

Epidemiology and Etiology

What age group presents with pain disorder?	Fourth to fifth decade
What gender presents with pain disorder more frequently?	2:1 female to male ratio
What disorders are more common in relatives of individuals with pain disorder?	Depression, pain disorders, substance-related disorders
What is a theoretical benefit of having pain disorder?	Assumption of the sick role alleviates psychological conflicts.
! Can medical conditions exist in the setting of pain disorder?	Yes. However, psychological factors exaggerate the experience of pain in relation to the underlying medical condition.

Diagnosis

! What are the *DSM-IV* diagnostic characteristics of pain disorder?	• Severe pain in one or more anatomic sites • Pain impairs functioning • Psychological factors affect pain onset, severity, exacerbation, and maintenance • Symptoms are unintentional • Other psychiatric conditions do not better account for the pain
! How does pain disorder differ from pain presenting in factitious disorder or malingering?	Pain disorder symptoms are *not* intentionally produced.
What subtypes of pain disorder exist?	• Associated with psychological factors or psychological factors and medical conditions • Acute (less than 6 months) or chronic
What medical conditions are most common in "pain disorder associated with medical conditions"?	Malignancies, musculoskeletal conditions, neuropathies

What is the differential diagnosis for pain disorders?

Factitious disorder, general medical condition, somatization disorder, malingering

Treatment

! **What pharmacologic interventions prove useful in treatment of pain disorder?**

Detoxification from pain medications or other drugs

What pharmacologic options have shown some benefits for pain disorder in patients?

- Tricyclic antidepressants
- SNRIs (eg, duloxetine [Cymbalta] and venlafaxine [Effexor])
- Monoamine oxidase inhibitors in combination with nonpharmacologic modalities
- Selective serotonin reuptake inhibitors

What lifestyle changes are recommended for patients with pain disorder?

Resume normal daily activities

What supportive measures exist for the treatment of pain disorder?

- Encouraging the patient to subscribe to a sense of personal commitment in allaying symptoms of pain
- Counseling on learning how to manage pain behaviorally
- Psychotherapy aimed at resolving underlying psychological conflicts
- Relaxation techniques
- Biofeedback

HYPOCHONDRIASIS

What is hypochondriasis?

Preoccupation with fear of disease and conviction that subtle bodily perceptions are manifestations of severe pathology

Epidemiology and Etiology

What age group presents with hypochondriasis?

Middle to late age

What gender presents with hypochondriasis more frequently?	Equal among males and females
What are predisposing factors for developing hypochondriasis?	• Parental attitudes toward disease • Personal past history of disease • Low socioeconomic class
What is a common psychodynamic explanation for hypochondriasis?	Displaced anxiety

Diagnosis

! **What is the core manifestation of hypochondriasis?**	Fear of having a disease stemming from misinterpreted bodily symptoms
! **How do hypochondriacs respond to medical evaluation of their complaints?**	Resistant to believing that extensive medical workups show no true pathology
! **How do hypochondriacs respond to reassurance provided by medical professionals?**	Poorly, often questioning physicians' credentials or seeking another opinion
! **How long must symptoms exist for the diagnosis of hypochondriasis to be made?**	At least 6 months
! **According to the *DSM-IV*, how must the symptoms be unique from other psychiatric disorders in the diagnosis of hypochondriasis?**	• Must not be delusional in nature • Must not be restricted to a concern about appearance as in body dysmorphic disorder • Must not be better explained by depression, obsessive-compulsive disorder, anxiety, separation disorder, or another somatoform disorder
What subtype of hypochondriasis exists?	With poor insight
How is this subtype characterized?	Some delusional aspect is present in that patients are not able to recognize that their preoccupations with having a serious disease are excessive in some way.
What is the differential diagnosis of hypochondriasis?	General medical conditions, delusional disorder (somatic type), normal health concerns

What two psychiatric conditions most frequently accompany the diagnosis of hypochondriasis?	Major depressive disorder and generalized anxiety disorder

Treatment

! **What complications may arise from hypochondriasis?**	Inherent risks associated with repeated diagnostic testing
What is the clinical course of hypochondriasis?	Waxing and waning according to psychological stressors
What is the most important step in management of hypochondriasis?	Obtaining and clearly documenting a complete psychosocial history
What is the most effective long-term treatment strategy for hypochondriasis?	Providing psychiatric care in conjunction with regular appointments with a primary care physician who conducts complete physical examinations as normally recommended

BODY DYSMORPHIC DISORDER

! **What is body dysmorphic disorder?**	Preoccupation with a specific blemish of physical appearance in a normally appearing individual

Epidemiology and Etiology

What age group most commonly presents with body dysmorphic disorder?	Adolescents
What gender presents with body dysmorphic disorder more frequently?	Equal among males and females
What are predisposing factors for developing body dysmorphic disorder?	• Parental attitudes toward appearance • Cultural or societal attitudes toward appearance • Low self-esteem
To which fields of medicine do patients with body dysmorphic disorder typically present?	Primary care physicians, plastic surgeons, dermatologists

Diagnosis

! **According to the *DSM-IV,* what is the core manifestation of body dysmorphic disorder?**	Self-perception of ugliness or obsession with some imagined physical flaw
! **Can a physical defect actually exist in a patient with body dysmorphic disorder?**	Yes, but the defect is exaggerated in its contribution to deformity.
How may these obsessive thoughts be manifested in behaviors?	Repetitive activities such as picking at the skin, staring into a mirror, or seeking approval from others regarding appearance
! **How must these preoccupying thoughts affect one's life in order to satisfy the *DSM-IV* criteria for body dysmorphic disorder?**	Impairment of function in daily activity including avoidance of social situations due to fear of exposing the exaggerated physical flaw to others
What key psychiatric disorder must be differentiated from body dysmorphic disorder?	Preoccupation with body image due to bulimia or anorexia nervosa
What is the differential diagnosis of body dysmorphic disorder?	Anorexia nervosa, social phobia, gender identity disorder, avoidant personality disorder, normal concerns about appearance (especially transient as in normal adolescent development), delusional disorder (somatic type), other somatization disorders

Treatment

! **What is an important initial step in management of body dysmorphic disorder?**	Evaluating the patient for comorbid psychiatric conditions such as depression and anxiety that may be especially amenable to pharmacologic or psychotherapeutic interventions
What specific treatment may be most beneficial for body dysmorphic disorder?	Individual or group cognitive-behavioral therapy aimed at psychosocial functioning and body image
! **What is the indication for use of antipsychotic medication in body dysmorphic disorder?**	When the preoccupation becomes delusional in character

! **What is the indication for use of selective serotonin reuptake inhibitors in body dysmorphic disorder?**	When mood disorders coexist

FACTITIOUS DISORDERS

! **What are factitious disorders?**	Disorders occurring when an individual willfully creates signs or symptoms of medical or psychiatric disease to assume the sick role
Are factitious disorders a type of somatoform disorder?	No, these entities are distinct categories of disorders in the *DSM-IV.*
What is the most severe type of factitious disorder?	Munchausen syndrome variant

Epidemiology and Etiology

What gender presents with factitious disorders more frequently?	Male, often health care workers
! **What is the most common presentation of Munchausen syndrome variant?**	Middle aged, unmarried, unemployed male feigning symptoms and signs of illness severe enough to be hospitalized several times while moving from one medical center to another to avoid discovery
! **What does a patient gain from creating signs or symptoms of disease in order to assume the sick role?**	Benefits of the sick role may include receiving careful attention, nurturing, and support from health care professionals.

Diagnosis

What elements of history and examination are suggestive of factitious disorders?	• Vague or inconsistent medical history conveyed in a highly guarded manner • Surprising familiarity for medical terminology or procedures in non-health care professionals due to involvement in health care • History of repeatedly moving from one health care setting to another • History in excess of physical findings • Evidence of multiple surgical scars on examination

! What are the *DSM-IV* diagnostic criteria for factitious disorder?	• Physical or psychological signs or symptoms are intentionally produced or faked. • The motivation for the behavior is to assume the sick role. • Secondary gains or external incentives for the behavior are absent.
What may result as a by-product of feigning illness in factitious disorders?	Iatrogenic injury including drug intoxication or physical trauma
What subtypes of factitious disorders exist?	With psychological signs and symptoms, physical signs and symptoms, or a combination
! What is factitious disorder by proxy?	Producing signs and symptoms of illness in another individual
! What is a common example of factitious disorder by proxy?	"Munchausen syndrome by proxy:" A person (most often a mother) deliberately causes injury or illness to another person (most often her child), usually to gain attention or some other benefit.
! How must Munchausen syndrome by proxy be treated by health care workers?	The previous example of a parent deliberately causing markers of illness in her child is a form of child abuse and *must* be reported.
What is the most common personality disorder associated with factitious disorder?	Borderline
What is the differential diagnosis of factitious disorder?	Malingering, actual general medical conditions, somatoform disorders
! How can factitious disorder be differentiated from other somatoform disorders?	Signs and symptoms are consciously produced by the patient.
! How can factitious disorder be differentiated from malingering?	Signs and symptoms are consciously produced to assume the sick role, not to obtain external incentives.
When is the onset of factitious disorder?	Adulthood, often following a hospitalization or health care experience
How can the course of factitious disorder be characterized?	Chronic, often switching between health care systems separated by geography

Treatment

! **How does a patient with factitious disorder respond to confrontation about the possibility that they are simulating illness?**	Patients are extremely resistant when confronted and may express anger and denial even in the face of overwhelming evidence that their signs and symptoms are intentionally produced. Often these patients will leave the health care setting by signing out AMA (against medical advice) or eloping from the emergency room.
How can further iatrogenic complications be avoided?	Explicit documentation and communication between health care providers as to the false nature of illness
How should factitious disorders be managed?	Evaluation and appropriate treatment of other comorbid conditions, psychotherapy, and confrontation in appropriate patients once rapport has been established in the doctor-patient relationship

MALINGERING

! **What is malingering?**	Purposeful creation of signs and symptoms of illness in order to gain external incentives such as money, medications, successful litigation, or excuse from responsibilities

Etiology and Epidemiology

Is malingering a mental illness?	No. Malingering is listed in the *DSM-IV* as "Other Conditions That May Be a Focus of Clinical Attention"
What gender presents with malingering more frequently?	Male

In what four circumstances should malingering be suspected?

1. Litigation is involved.
2. Clinical presentation is out of proportion to physical examination or testing.
3. Patient exhibits difficulty in adhering to a medical regimen or participating in diagnostic testing.
4. Underlying antisocial personality disorder.

How can the onset of malingering be characterized?

Onset is directly related to the availability of environmental incentives.

Diagnosis

What are the two essential components of malingering?

1. Signs and symptoms of illness are consciously created by the patient in the absence of true pathology.
2. Ultimate goal of such behavior is to obtain some external incentive.

Treatment

! **How can malingering behavior be terminated?**

Remove the external incentive

What concepts are important in dealing with malingering?

- Maintaining confidentiality
- Using a nonjudgmental approach to confronting the patient
- Demonstrating willingness to explore possible underlying psychosocial issues that may be contributing to malingering through psychotherapy

CLINICAL VIGNETTES

A 38-year-old white man presents to the ER with fever and "swollen arms." The patient was in his usual state of health until he developed a fever of 102.5°F and his right arm became red and edematous. He is vague when discussing his past medical history. He denies any alcohol or substance abuse. On examination, he is febrile, tachycardic, and anxious. Pus can be expressed from multiple venipuncture sites on his right arm with surrounding erythema, and induration. On trying to obtain old medical records it becomes evident that he has visited several medical centers across the Midwest. When questioned about his previous hospital visits and the nature of the venipuncture sites, he becomes extremely angry and yells, "What does it matter? Can't you see I am sick?" How can this disorder be differentiated from other somatoform disorders?

In factitious disorder, signs and symptoms are consciously produced to obtain the sick role; the history of multiple hospital visits separated by geography and infection with an obvious, self-inflicted source suggests the diagnosis of factitious disorder. Patients afflicted with this disorder may have anger against authority figures or issues of dependency, but most often they have a need to assume the "sick role." Their purpose in assuming this role is to receive nurturing, support, and attention from health care professionals. In comparison to other somatoform disorders, signs and symptoms are **consciously** produced by the patient to obtain the **sick role** and not for external incentives.

A 31-year-old woman with a history of a prior caesarian section for a triplet pregnancy presents to her family physician with an inability to enjoy sexual intercourse. Over the last 2 years she has had difficulty becoming sexually aroused with her partner of 10 years. In addition, she reports experiencing nausea; frequent diarrhea; headache; muscular pain in her legs, neck, and back; and numbness in her fingers. She thinks that her mother had experienced similar symptoms when she was younger. Her father has lived in her home over the past 3 years while dying of pancreatic cancer. What is the ideal approach to managing this disorder?

Manage somatization disorder by providing psychological support through a therapeutic relationship; in the absence of a medical cause, the existence of a sexual symptom, at least four pain symptoms, at least two GI symptoms, and at least one pseudoneurologic symptom all beginning before the age of 30 and lasting for at least 2 years is suggestive of somatization disorder. This disorder is more common in females, lower socioeconomic class, and those with family history of illness. The symptoms are not consciously produced by the patient. The ideal approach to managing this disorder involves commitment to developing a therapeutic doctor-patient relationship and providing psychological support in the form of regular follow-up visits focused on psychotherapeutics instead of further medical workup.

A 25-year-old white woman presents to her primary care physician with intractable nausea over the last year. Nothing seems to alleviate the nausea. She has tried antiemetics and a complete change in her diet to no avail. She also complains of headache and pain in her legs and arms. Her menstrual cycles have been regular and a pregnancy test is negative. Her vitals signs and physical examination are normal. Further workup reveals no abnormalities in electrolytes, complete blood count (CBC), endocrine studies, and viral liters. All imaging to this point has been negative. What is the most likely diagnosis?

Undifferentiated somatoform disorder; with a negative medical workup and multiple somatic complaints, a somatoform disorder is likely. Because these symptoms are fewer and of shorter duration than those required for the diagnosis of somatization disorder, the diagnosis of undifferentiated somatoform disorder is more appropriate. Once medical causes have been ruled out, the treatment of undifferentiated somatoform disorder does not differ from that of somatization disorder.

A 41-year-old man presents to his primary care physician with back pain. He reports that he has been afflicted by back pain for years but now it has become intolerable. He works as a plumber and says that he cannot imagine having to work in this condition. He claims that the only thing that has helped him in the past has been Percocet. He asks for a prescription and a note for work so that he can file for disability. He has had no bowel or bladder trouble. On examination, his back is mildly tender to palpation with no sensory loss and negative straight leg raise testing. He walks with an exaggerated limp while clutching his flank. What concepts are important in the treatment of this condition?

Malingering—remove the external incentive; although this patient may have true back pain, his presentation is out of proportion to the relatively benign physical examination. This presentation, in the context of external incentives such as pain medication and being excused from work, is highly suggestive of malingering. The therapeutic approach to such a patient should be nonjudgmental, confidential, and should offer the patient an opportunity for psychotherapy that may reveal underlying psychosocial issues driving the malingering behavior.

A 42-year-old woman presents to the ED with a "paralyzed leg." She was in her normal state of health until this morning when suddenly she could not move her left leg. This has never happened to her before. She has a history of hypertension treated with hydrochlorothiazide but otherwise has no medical problems. She has no history of psychiatric disease. On examination, her blood pressure is mildly elevated. Neurologic examination reveals normal strength and range of motion in all extremities except the left leg. She is unable to lift the left leg off the bed. Normal tone is present in the leg with no sign of flaccidity. With help, she can swing her legs over the bed and stand on both feet. Psychiatric examination finds no mood or anxiety symptoms. She does reveal that she was sexually abused as a child and her husband recently lost his job. She has two children who are doing well at college. What is the treatment of this disorder?

Treat conversion disorder with reassurance, psychotherapy, and suggestive techniques; pseudoneurologic symptoms such as paresis in the context of psychosocial stressors suggest the diagnosis of conversion disorder. The fact that she cannot move her leg but is able to stand on it rules out true paresis. This disorder is more common in women, especially those with a history of sexual abuse and current psychosocial stressors. After general medical causes are ruled out, patients can be treated using a variety of suggestive techniques including hypnosis and psychotherapy. Since the patient is not consciously producing the symptom, she should not be confronted about its production. In most cases the patient is responsive to suggestive techniques or the disorder is self-limiting.

A 56-year-old Asian woman with a history of hypothyroidism presents to her family physician with a 3-month history of severe pain in her neck and legs. Her job as an administrative assistant has been extremely demanding since she was hired 5 months ago. She is recently divorced and her recent attempts at dating other people have been unsuccessful. She has been taking Percocet without much pain relief. She has been out of work for 3 days because her pain has bothered her so much. She reports no history of trauma. Physical examination reveals diffuse tenderness to palpation over the back of her neck and the back of her legs without any loss in sensation or motor strength. There is no joint swelling or erythema of her joints and her antinuclear antibody screen is negative. What is the nature of her pain and how should it be treated?

Pain disorder—pain is unintentional and should be treated with detoxification of pain medications, resumption of normal activity, behavioral techniques, and psychotherapy; severe pain in multiple anatomic sites, psychological impact of a stressful job and recent disarray in personal life, and impairment in function preventing her from going to work suggest the diagnosis of pain disorder. The pain seen in pain disorder is unintentional in nature. General medical conditions, such as autoimmune causes in this case, need to be ruled out before the diagnosis is made. Treatment of pain disorder involves detoxifying patients from pain medications, encouraging the resumption of their normal daily activities, psychotherapy, and educating the patient on behavioral techniques effective in dealing with pain. The use of tricyclic antidepressants (TCAs), monoamine oxidase inhibitors (MAOIs), and SS/NRIs has shown benefit in some patients with pain disorder.

A 29-year-old mother brings her 3-year-old child to the ER after the child "passed out." At home, the 3-year-old is normally very active and has been developmentally normal with regular visits to her family physician until a year ago when the mother and son moved four times within three different states. The mother, who works as a nurse, appears very anxious and concerned about the health of her son. On examination, the child is lethargic and pale. Fingerstick measures glucose of 45. Lab work shows increased insulin levels and decreased C-peptide levels. What is the diagnosis?

Factitious disorder by proxy—in this case it is a form of child abuse and must be reported! The cause of the child's hypoglycemia is most likely iatrogenic. Hypoglycemia in the setting of high insulin levels and low C-peptide levels is suggestive of iatrogenic exogenous insulin administration as exogenous insulin preparations do not contain C-peptide. The diagnosis of factitious disorder by proxy is appropriate in this case as the signs and symptoms of illness in the son were produced by the mother. Frequently, individuals with this diagnosis are familiar with the medical field in some capacity.

A 62-year-old man with a past history of basal cell skin cancer presents to his dermatologist with a dark spot on his arm. This is his 15th visit to a dermatologist over the last 6 months. Each visit he has pointed out a different dark spot on his arm. He has switched dermatologists three times because they have reassured him that each spot is not suspicious of cancer. On examination, the spot is less than 3 mm, perfectly round with regular borders, and light brown in color without any area of darker pigmentation. He remarks that he is terrified of dying from skin cancer. What complications may arise as a result of this disorder?

Complications in hypochondriasis may arise from repeated tests or procedures; this man's preoccupation with fear of skin cancer and conviction that subtle bodily perceptions are manifestations of severe pathology suggest the diagnosis of hypochondriasis. Personal past history of disease, such as basal cell carcinoma in this man, is a predisposing factor. Patients with hypochondriasis often doubt the credentials of their physicians or seek second opinions. Because of the frequency and conviction with which they present to health care facilities, multiple diagnostic tests are usually conducted. The most likely complication of hypochondriasis stems from the risks of the tests or diagnostic procedures. Gathering a sound psychosocial history and documentation of hypochondriasis may help to avoid future unnecessary testing.

A 15-year-old girl presents to her family physician with her mother because of her "huge nose." Her mother reports that her daughter has recently been skipping school and not attending after school activities or volleyball practice but has been jogging by herself twice a day. The girl describes her nose as "gargantuan," "bigger than everyone else's at school," and "embarrassing." She requests a referral to a plastic surgeon so that her nose can be "fixed." Age at menarche was 12 and her menstrual cycles have been regular without any missed periods. On examination, the girl is well appearing, thin, and her nose appears the size of most other girls her age. What is the indication for use of SSRIs in this disorder?[1]

Mood disorders comorbid with body dysmorphic disorder; preoccupation with a specific aspect of physical appearance in a normally appearing adolescent is suggestive of body dysmorphic disorder. Patients with this disorder present most frequently to primary care physicians, dermatologists, or plastic surgeons. This patient manifests fear of exposing the exaggerated physical flaw to others in her avoidant behavior. Although she has been exercising more regularly, the lack of any change in her menstrual cycles does not support a diagnosis of anorexia, an important differential diagnosis. Patients with body dysmorphic disorder must be evaluated for comorbid psychiatric conditions, especially mood disorders, as they may be amenable to pharmacologic intervention such as an SSRI.

CHAPTER 9

Sleep Disorders

EPIDEMIOLOGY AND ETIOLOGY

Define primary sleep disorders.

Disorders that occur as a result of disturbances in one's sleep-wake cycle

Define secondary sleep disorders.

Disorders that occur as a result of other medical or mental conditions (eg, bipolar disorder, substance dependence)

! **Differentiate parasomnias from dyssomnias.**

- Dyssomnias refer to perturbations in the amount or quality of sleep
- Parasomnias refer to abnormal physiology or behavior in sleep
- Both terms fall under the broader category of primary sleep disorders.

What are the subtypes of dyssomnias?

- Primary insomnia
- Primary hypersomnia
- Narcolepsy
- Breathing-related disorders
- Circadian rhythm sleep disorder
- Dyssomnia not otherwise specified

What are the subtypes of parasomnias?

- Nightmare disorder
- Sleep terror disorder
- Sleepwalking disorder
- Parasomnia not otherwise specified

! What is the normal sleep cycle, and what are the associated electroencephalogram (EEG) wave forms?

- Nonrapid eye movement (NREM) sleep (75% of sleep cycle)
    - Eyes closed—awake (**alpha waves**)
    - Stage 1—very light sleep (**loss of alpha waves**)
    - Stage 2—light sleep (**sleep spindles and k-complexes**)
    - Stage 3-4—Slow wave sleep (**delta waves**)
- REM sleep (25% of sleep cycle)
    - Cycles occur approximately every 90 minutes and last around 30 minutes
    - Dreaming
    - Erections, atonia
    - EEC shows "**saw tooth" waves**

What stage of sleep, if decreased, will make a person feel the most "tired"?

Slow wave (or "deep") sleep (stage 3-4)

Does amount of REM sleep increase, decrease, or stay the same with age?

Decrease

What part of the hypothalamus is thought to play a major role in the sleep-wake cycle or circadian rhythm?

Suprachiasmatic nucleus (SCN)

What psychiatric disorders are associated with sleep disorders?

- Depression
- Anxiety disorders
- Posttraumatic stress disorder (PTSD)
- Schizophrenia
- Substance abuse (especially alcohol)

DIAGNOSIS AND TREATMENT

Primary Insomnia

What is primary insomnia?

Difficulty initiating or maintaining sleep for at least 1 month. This results in excessive daytime sleepiness, which can impair daily functioning.

How is primary insomnia diagnosed?

It is generally a diagnosis of exclusion that is made once other medical, substance-related, and psychiatric etiologies have been ruled out.

What concurrent conditions will exacerbate primary insomnia?

Anxiety, especially related to the insomnia itself

How is primary insomnia treated?

- Improve sleep hygiene (first line)
- Pharmacotherapy (for short-term usage)

What is sleep hygiene?

Sleep hygiene refers to good sleep habits or rituals that are conducive to helping one initiate and maintain sleep throughout the night.

List some examples of good sleep hygiene.

- Maintain a regular sleep cycle (same time to get in bed to sleep and wake up in the morning)
- Keep the room quiet
- Limit caffeine, nicotine, and alcohol intake, especially before bedtime
- Use the bed and bedroom primarily for the three "S's": sleep, sickness, and sex
- Eat a light snack before bedtime
- Avoid daytime naps
- If you are unable to fall asleep after 30 minutes, get out of bed and engage in a relaxing activity (eg, reading) for some time before coming back to bed. The key is to associate the bed with sleep, not frustration.

What drugs may be useful in the short-term treatment of this condition?

Diphenhydramine (Benadryl), trazodone (Desyrel), zolpidem (Ambien), zaleplon (Sonata), eszopiclone (Lunesta). Diphenhydramine (Benadryl) and trazodone (Desyrel) should be tried first because they are less likely to be habit-forming.

! Is alcohol a good treatment for insomnia?

No. Alcohol does lead to a more rapid induction of sleep, and it also increases NREM sleep and reduces REM sleep during the first portion of the night. However, it is metabolized rapidly and blood concentrations are negligible by the middle of the night, which results in withdrawal symptoms such as shallow sleep with multiple awakenings, REM rebound associated with nightmares or vivid dreams, sweating, and general activation. Therefore, although alcohol may be effective in sleep induction, it impairs sleep during the second half of the night and can lead to a reduction in overall sleep time.

Primary Hypersomnia

Define primary hypersomnia.	Excessive sleepiness for at least 1 month, not attributable to other medical, psychiatric, substance-related, or preexisting sleep conditions. This disorder usually results in a decline in daily functioning.
What are the common complaints of patients with primary hypersomnia?	Excessive, nonrefreshing sleep, and/or difficult awakenings
How is primary hypersomnia diagnosed?	Polysomnographic testing (not by patient reports)
What is the differential diagnosis of primary hypersomnia?	Klein-Levine syndrome
What is Klein-Levine syndrome?	Affected patients experience hypersomnia for the majority of the day accompanied by episodes of inappropriate behavior (sexual or otherwise) and compulsive eating.
Klein-Levin syndrome typically presents in what patient demographic?	Adolescent boys
How is Klein-Levin syndrome treated?	It is treated with amphetamines, selective serotonin reuptake inhibitors (SSRIs), or monoamine oxidase inhibitors (MAOIs).
What is the treatment for primary hypersomnia?	Stimulants (eg, amphetamines) are first line, but SSRIs and MAOIs may be effective as well.

Narcolepsy

What is narcolepsy?	A dyssomnia characterized by repeated episodes of sudden REM sleep during wakefulness for at least 3 months
! **What is the classic tetrad of narcolepsy?**	1. *Cataplexy:* episodes of loss of skeletal muscle tone leading to collapse, sometimes brought on by laughter or strong emotion 2. *Sleep paralysis:* brief paralysis upon wakening 3. *Short REM latency:* short period of time from initiation of sleep to first REM cycle 4. *Sleep hallucinations:* hypnagogic and/or hypnopompic

! Differentiate the two major types of sleep hallucinations.

Hypnagogic hallucinations occur as the patient is falling asleep.
- **Think: g = going to sleep**

Hypnopompic occur as the patient is waking.
- **Think: p = perking up**

Which gender is predisposed to narcolepsy?

It affects men and women equally.

In what age group is the onset of narcolepsy most common?

Young adulthood

What is the most definitive test used to diagnose narcolepsy?

Sleep latency test

In narcoleptics, what is the quality of their "regular" nighttime sleep?

Poor

How is narcolepsy treated?

Stimulants such as methylphenidate (Ritalin), dextroamphetamine (Adderall), or modafinil (Provigil) are used along with timed naps to treat the sleep attacks. SSRIs or tricyclic antidepressants (TCAs) are used for cataplexy.

Breathing-Related Sleep Disorders

What are breathing-related sleep disorders (BRSDs)?

Excessive daytime sleepiness or recurrent disruption of normal sleep secondary to sleep apnea or hypoventilation

What percentage of the adult population is affected by BRSDs?

~10%

What are predisposing factors for this condition?

Male gender and obesity

What other conditions or symptoms are associated with BRSDs?

Headaches, depression, and pulmonary hypertension

What are the two major types of sleep apnea?

Obstructive and central

Which type of sleep apnea is associated with snoring?

Obstructive sleep apnea (OSA)

Describe OSA.

Apnea resulting from collapse of the upper airway resulting in disrupted sleep. It also results in hypoxemia, hypercapnia, and hypertension.

What are risk factors for OSA?

- Obesity
- Male gender
- Large neck circumference
- History of airway surgery
- Deviated nasal septum
- Large tongue
- Retrognathia (mandible is posterior to its normal position in relation to the maxillae)

How is OSA treated?

- Weight loss
- Continuous positive airway pressure (CPAP)
- Surgery (second-line treatment)

What is central sleep apnea (CSA)?

Apnea during sleep that results from failure of the central nervous system to activate the muscles of respiration

How is CSA diagnosed?

Documenting cessation of breathing for 10–120 seconds, with at least 5 such episodes of apnea per hour. This can be done during a sleep study.

What is the treatment for CSA?

Mechanical ventilation, commonly with BiPAP (bilevel positive airway pressure)

How does CPAP differ from BiPAP?

CPAP delivers a constant pressure. BiPAP's pressure varies with the patient's breathing.

Circadian Rhythm Sleep Disorder

What is a circadian rhythm sleep disorder?

Sleep disorder resulting from a mismatch between the hypothalamic sleep-wake cycle and the environmental demands on one's sleep-wake cycle

What are the common symptoms of a circadian rhythm sleep disorder?

Hypersomnia, insomnia, and fatigue

What are some subtypes of circadian rhythm sleep disorder?

- Jet lag
- Shiftwork
- Advanced or delayed sleep phase

How is jet lag usually treated?

Jet lag usually resolves without treatment after 2-7 days.

What treatments can be effective in lessening the severity of symptoms associated with jet lag?

- Attempt to synchronize one's clock to the new time zone with naps or staying awake longer than usual
- Short course of benzodiazepines as sleep aids
- Multiple studies have found that melatonin, taken close to the target bedtime at the destination, decreased jet lag.

Does traveling east advance your sleep cycle or delay the cycle?

Traveling east will advance the sleep cycle, whereas traveling west will delay it.

Who is most prone to shift work sleep disorder?

People who alternate between working day shifts and night shifts (such as residents!)

What are delayed sleep phase disorders?

The patient's sleep-wake cycle is shifted relative to conventional rest-activity periods, for example, "night owls."

What is a treatment for delayed sleep phase disorder?

Light therapy

Nightmare Disorder

In what phase of the sleep cycle do nightmares occur?

REM sleep. More often than not, the nightmares occur in the second half of the sleep period.

When in a patient's lifetime is the onset of this disorder most common?

During childhood

Is the patient usually oriented after awakening from a nightmare?

Yes

How is nightmare disorder treated?

Usually, this disorder does not require treatment, but TCAs have been effective in shortening REM sleep and hence lessening the frequency of nightmares.

Sleep Terror Disorder

Describe sleep terror disorder.	Patients will awaken suddenly and be in a state of intense fear and anxiety. They may experience tachycardia and diaphoresis. They are unable to be comforted or consoled during these episodes and they remain **amnestic** throughout. They are generally unable to recall the event when awakened in the morning.
What demographic is most susceptible to sleep terrors?	Children
What phase of sleep do these sleep terrors occur?	Stage 3 and 4 (NREM) sleep
While sleep terrors are usually self-limited, how can they be treated?	Benzodiazepines at bedtime may be effective by decreasing delta sleep (stage 3-4).

Sleepwalking Disorder

Describe sleepwalking disorder.	Episodes of getting out of bed and walking, generally occurring during the first third of a night's sleep. **Patients have a blank stare, can be difficult to awaken, and may be unresponsive to others.** Most episodes end with patients safely returning to their bed and falling back asleep. **If the patient is awakened during an episode, they are generally disoriented.**
What age is the peak prevalence for sleepwalking?	12 years old
What is the best treatment for sleepwalking?	Maintaining a safe environment so as to minimize injury during a sleep walking episode

CLINICAL VIGNETTES

A 19-year-old female college student reports occasionally falling sleep in the middle of the day. This occurs even when she is with her girlfriends watching their favorite daytime soap opera. She also says that she is always tired in the mornings before class despite going to bed at a reasonable hour. She reports seeing the image of her dead cousin flying above her bed just before she falls asleep. She has come to your office today because when she awoke this morning, she was unable to move despite being alert to her surroundings. This lasted only 20 seconds, but she was very upset by the episode. What is the most likely diagnosis and how would you proceed with treatment?

Narcolepsy; the patient exhibits some classic symptoms of narcolepsy: sudden sleep attacks during the day, cataplexy, and hypnagogic hallucinations. (Remember: hypnagogic—going to sleep; hypnopompic—perking up.) Narcolepsy in this case would likely be treated with timed daytime naps and stimulants such as methylphenidate (Ritalin), dextroamphetamine (Adderall), or modafinil (Provigil).

A 9-year-old boy comes into his parents' room in the middle of the night. He is crying and screaming and when asked what the problem is, he responds simply with more crying. His parents try to console him, but he remains upset until he soon returns to bed and falls back asleep. In the morning, the boy has no recollection of the event. His parents comment that this sort of episode has been happening for months. What is the diagnosis?

Sleep terror disorder; the patient awakes upset, is unable to be consoled, and is unable to recall the event. All of these features are suggestive of a sleep terror.

A 19-year-old man reports "not being able to sleep." He reports no other symptoms, denies excessive daytime sleepiness, and states that his tossing and turning in bed is a problem nearly every night. Since he is a young man, he has relatively little medical history, and he is not taking any prescribed medications. You cannot give him a diagnosis at this visit and he returns 6 weeks later with the same complaints and now is concerned because his schoolwork is suffering. What other test might you order?

Toxicology screen; substance abuse is a common cause of sleep disorders, specifically insomnia. This patient should be screened for multiple drugs, including alcohol and cocaine. However, prior to ordering a toxicology screen, the physician must take a detailed drug history. By identifying drug use and offering the patient help and treatment, he may be able to get over this current insomnia and also avoid many deleterious health consequences in the future.

A 47-year-old man returns to your primary care office for his yearly examination. You are currently treating him for hypertension and hypercholesterolemia. Despite your repeated urgings for your patient to lose weight, he returns 20 lb heavier than last year. As you complete the interview and physical examination, he complains that he has been experiencing an occasional headache. On walking your patient out to the waiting room, you see his wife waiting there for him. When she sees you she immediately says to her husband: "You told the doctor about the snoring... RIGHT!?" The patient then proceeds to explain that his wife has recently noticed him snoring and that she thinks that he stops breathing during sleep. What is the most likely diagnosis?

Obstructive sleep apnea (OSA); the patient has the typical overweight habitus observed in individuals with OSA. These patients are prone to OSA as excessive body fat (around their necks) tends to collapse their upper airway when the patients are supine during sleep. This is the same mechanism that can produce snoring.

A 59-year-old man in excellent physical condition and with no significant past medical history presents to your office with complaints of daytime sleepiness. He reports nearly falling asleep while driving to your office. You order a sleep study that shows an average of seven apneic episodes per hour, each lasting between 20 and 30 seconds. Does this man meet the diagnostic criteria for sleep apnea? If so, what type? What other disease is associated with this type of sleep apnea?

Yes, he meets the criteria for central sleep apnea (CSA): at least five episodes of apnea per hour, each lasting between 10 and 120 seconds. CSA is associated with heart failure, although it appears unlikely that the patient in this case would have heart failure given his (lack of) medical history.

A 29-year-old woman presents to you with the complaint of insomnia. You discuss the concepts of sleep hygiene with her (eg, using the bed primarily for sleep, sickness, and sex; maintaining a regular sleep schedule; avoiding alcohol and caffeine; etc) and ask her to follow up in a few weeks time. At her follow-up visit, she states that she still has difficulty falling asleep. What treatment should you offer?

Medications with less potential for abuse, like diphenhydramine (Benadryl) and trazodone (Desyrel), should be tried first. If these do not work, non-benzodiazepine hypnotics (eg, zolpidem [Ambien], zaleplon [Sonata], eszopiclone [Lunesta]) can be tried. Zolpidem (Ambien) and zaleplon (Sonata) have shorter half-lives and are better for sleep induction. Eszopiclone (Lunesta) has a longer half-life and is better for sleep maintenance.

A 9-year-old boy comes into his parents' room in the middle of the night. He is crying and screaming and when asked what the problem is, he responds simply with more crying. His parents try to console him, but he remains upset until he soon returns to bed and falls back asleep. In the morning, the boy has no recollection of the event. His parents comment that this sort of episode has been happening for months. What is the diagnosis?

Sleep terror disorder; the patient awakes upset, is unable to be consoled, and is unable to recall the event. All of these features are suggestive of a sleep terror.

CHAPTER 10

Substance-Related Disorders

INTRODUCTION

! **How is substance abuse defined by the *DSM-IV* (*Diagnostic and Statistical Manual of Mental Disorders, Fourth Edition*)?**

A pattern of substance use that causes clinically significant impairment for at least 12 months with at least one of the following:

- Failure to fulfill social or professional obligations
- The use of substances in physically hazardous situations (eg, driving while under the influence of alcohol)
- Recurrent legal problems stemming from substance use
- Continued use despite surrounding personal problems related to the use

Think of the 3 **Cs: compulsive** use, loss of **control**, and **continued** use despite adverse consequences

! How is substance dependence defined by the *DSM-IV*?

A pattern of substance use leading to at least three of the following over a 12-month period:

- *Tolerance*: the need for increased amounts of a substance in order to achieve the desired effect or a markedly decreased effect with the same amount of substance
- *Withdrawal*: the development of characteristic symptoms due to cessation of use after prolonged usage of a substance
- Use of a substance in greater amounts or over a longer period of time than originally intended
- Persistent desire or wish to cut down or control substance use
- Spending significant time obtaining, using, or recovering from the substance
- Decreased social or professional activities due to substance use
- Continued use despite knowledge of significant physical, social, or psychological problems stemming from the substance use

ALCOHOL

Epidemiology and Etiology

Is alcohol an activating or inhibiting substance?

Alcohol activates gamma-aminobutyric acid (GABA) receptors (which are inhibitory ion channels) and hence results in central nervous system (CNS) inhibition or sedation.

What are the two major enzymes involved in alcohol (ethanol) metabolism?

Alcohol dehydrogenase and aldehyde dehydrogenase

Aldehyde dehydrogenase is commonly lacking or deficient in what ethnic group?

Asians

Deficiency in this enzyme leads to a buildup of what metabolite?

Acetylaldehyde

What are the physical manifestations of this enzyme deficiency after alcohol ingestion?

Flushing and nausea

What percentage of Americans can be classified as "alcoholics"?

7%-10%

What is the ratio of male:female prevalence of alcohol dependence?

4:1

Diagnosis

What is the CAGE Questionnaire?

A screening tool for alcoholism consisting of the following four questions. Two or more responses of "yes" are a positive result.

1. Have you ever wanted to **C**ut down on your drinking?
2. Have you ever felt **A**nnoyed by criticism of your drinking?
3. Have you ever felt **G**uilty about drinking?
4. Have you ever needed a drink as an **E**ye-opener?

What is one alcoholic drink?

One standard drink is equivalent to 12 ounces of beer, 5 ounces of wine, or 1.5 ounces of 80-proof spirits.

What is another quick way to screen for alcohol abuse?

Ask "how many times in the past year have you had (for men) 5 or more drinks/(for women) 4 or more drinks?" If the answer is 1 or more, ask "on average, how many days a week do you have an alcoholic drink, and on a typical drinking day, how many drinks do you have?"

What are the recommended maximum drinking limits?

According to the National Institute of Alcohol Abuse and Alcoholism, for healthy men up to age 65, no more than 4 drinks in a day and 14 drinks in a week, and for healthy women and men over age 65, no more than 3 drinks in a day and 7 drinks in a week.

What range of blood alcohol level (BAL) is considered the legal limit for intoxication in most states?

80-100 mg/dL

What BAL will lead to respiratory depression in most "nonalcoholic" drinkers?	400 mg/dL
! **In unresponsive or semiconscious patients who are suspected to have used alcohol, what intervention should be considered first?**	Intubation for airway protection
What are common reasons for presenting with alcohol intoxication?	Falls, blackouts, altercations, and accidents
What is the differential diagnosis of alcohol intoxication?	Hypoxia, hypoglycemia, other drug overdose/intoxication, ethylene glycol or methanol poisoning, hepatic encephalopathy, psychosis
! **What are some early physical signs of alcoholism?**	Palmar erythema, acne rosacea, hepatomegaly
! **What are some signs of advanced alcoholism?**	Jaundice, cirrhosis, ascites, testicular atrophy, gynecomastia, Dupuytren contractures
What are Dupuytren contractures?	Thickening and tightening of the palmar fascia leading to contracture of the digits, most commonly the 4th and 5th digits
What are feared complications from alcoholic cirrhosis?	Variceal bleeding and hepatic encephalopathy
What is a feared complication from drinking "moonshine"?	Improper distilling techniques can result in excessive levels of methanol in moonshine which may result in blindness.
! **What is Wernicke-Korsakoff syndrome?**	A neuropsychiatric complication of chronic alcohol abuse. It results from thiamine (vitamin B1) deficiency in alcoholics owing to their poor diet as opposed to a direct result of alcohol ingestion. Wernicke encephalopathy is the early manifestation, and Korsakoff syndrome is the later manifestation.
! **What is the classic triad of Wernicke encephalopathy?**	1. Nystagmus 2. Ataxia 3. Confusion

Is Wernicke encephalopathy reversible?	Yes, with the administration of thiamine. Standard dose is 100 mg IV.
! **What *must* be given to patients before standard fluid replacement therapy?**	Thiamine must be given prior to any IV fluids containing glucose. Since glucose depletes thiamine stores, it cannot be given in any form (including D5½ NS) before thiamine as it would exacerbate the patient's condition.
What other supplement should be given to suspected alcoholics along with thiamine?	Folate
! **If Wernicke encephalopathy goes untreated and progresses to Korsakoff syndrome, what are the classic symptoms?**	1. Anterograde amnesia 2. Confabulation
What is confabulation?	To fill in gaps in one's memory with fabrications that one believes to be facts
Is Korsakoff syndrome reversible?	It is chronic and irreversible in two-thirds of patients.
Damage to what thiamine-dependent cerebral structures are thought to lead to the memory deficits of Korsakoff syndrome?	The **mammillary bodies** of the hypothalamus and the dorsal medial nucleus of the thalamus
What are some abnormal labs that may be observed in alcoholics?	Elevated high-density lipoprotein (HDL), mean corpuscular volume (MCV), and transaminases. Decreased low-density lipoprotein (LDL).
Which transaminase is particularly elevated in alcoholics?	Aspartate aminotransferase (AST). **Think: "A S**cotch and **T**onic."
What is the pathophysiology of alcohol withdrawal?	Although not fully understood, it is believed that when long-term ethyl alcohol (EtOH) ingestion stops there is a surge of neuronal activity. The loss of GABA excitation leads to release of inhibition on glutamate and hence a subsequent surge of activity.
What are the signs and symptoms of alcohol withdrawal?	• *Minor*: tremor, irritability, insomnia, nausea, vomiting, hypertension, tachycardia • *Mild*: diaphoresis, disorientation, fever • *Severe*: delirium tremens (DTs), seizures

How long after a patient's last drink will withdrawal symptoms usually begin and how long will they last?	6-24 hours after last drink, lasting 5-7 days
Is alcohol withdrawal life threatening?	Yes
When are seizures generally seen in alcohol withdrawal?	24-48 hours after last drink
! **What are DTs?**	DTs are a severe form of alcohol withdrawal consisting of delirium, hallucinations, and autonomic hyperarousal in addition to other withdrawal symptoms.
What percentage of patients hospitalized with alcohol withdrawal will develop DTs?	Approximately 5%
What percentage of patients with DTs will die if they are not treated?	15%-20% mortality. Therefore, DTs should be considered a medical emergency.
! **When is the peak incidence of DTs in withdrawal patients?**	Most commonly occur within 72 hours after the last drink, but may occur up to 7-10 days after the last drink

Treatment

How is alcohol withdrawal treated?	Benzodiazepines such as lorazepam (Ativan) or chlordiazepoxide (Librium) along with supportive treatment with thiamine/folate and IV fluids
Should benzodiazepine therapy be started prior to signs of DTs?	Yes. They are used to prevent DTs as well as treat withdrawal.
What are treatments of alcohol dependence (in the nonacute setting)?	Self-help groups such as Alcoholics Anonymous (AA) or psychotherapy. Also pharmacologic therapy with disulfiram and naltrexone
What is the mechanism of action of disulfiram (Antabuse)?	Inhibition of aldehyde dehydrogenase leading to violent vomiting if ethanol is ingested. Standard dose is 250 mg daily.
What is the mechanism of action of naltrexone (Revia)?	Antagonism at opioid receptors

How can naltrexone (Revia) be helpful in treating alcohol dependence?

It significantly decreases rate, frequency, and severity of relapse; craving; and increases time to first drink. Standard dose is 50 mg daily.

What percentage of treated alcohol-dependent patients will relapse within 6 months?

50%

SEDATIVES AND HYPNOTICS

What two major classes of prescription medications are considered to be sedatives/hypnotics?

Benzodiazepines and barbiturates

What is the mechanism of action of benzodiazepines?

They activate GABA receptors and increase the frequency of opening of the chloride ion channel.

What is the mechanism of action of barbiturates?

They enhance activation of GABA-ergic chloride channels by increasing the duration of opening. **Think: "barbiturate" = increased duration.**

! Which class of sedatives are considered safer: benzodiazepines or barbiturates?

Benzodiazepines are considered safer as they are less likely to cause respiratory depression.

What are signs and symptoms of sedative/hypnotic intoxication?

Drowsiness, slurred speech, mood lability, confusion, ataxia, respiratory depression, and coma or death in extreme cases of overdose

How can sedative intoxication be differentiated from alcohol intoxication?

Signs and symptoms are similar. If alcohol cannot be detected on the breath, then serum or urine drug screens can be performed.

What substance is cross-tolerant with benzodiazepines and barbiturates (ie, patients with physiologic tolerance to one substance have tolerance to the others)?

Alcohol

! **What is the treatment for sedative overdose?**

- Airway maintenance
- Activated charcoal to prevent further gastrointestinal (GI) absorption
- Benzodiazepines: flumazenil
- Barbiturates: alkalinize urine with sodium bicarbonate to increase renal excretion

What is flumazenil?

A short-acting benzodiazepine antagonist

What is a side effect of flumazenil?

Seizures

Is withdrawal from short-acting or long-acting sedatives more dangerous?

Abrupt cessation of short-acting sedatives is more likely to cause severe withdrawal symptoms.

What are symptoms of sedative withdrawal?

Tremors, nausea, vomiting, tachycardia, weakness, anxiety, irritability, diaphoresis, hyperreflexia, orthostatic hypotension, seizures (can be life threatening)

What is the treatment for sedative withdrawal?

Scheduled, tapered dosing of a long-acting benzodiazepine or barbiturate such as diazepam (Valium) or phenobarbital. Anticonvulsants can be used for seizure control.

OPIATES

Epidemiology and Etiology

Give some examples of opiates.

Heroin, morphine, codeine, methadone, meperidine, dextromethorphan, and hydromorphone

What is the most common reason for prescription opiate use?

Pain control

What over-the-counter (OTC) medication containing an opiate is commonly used to "get high"?

Dextromethorphan, a lower potency opiate, is used in many cold remedies for its cough suppressant qualities.

What is the most common route of administration of opiates in addicts?

Intravenous

! **What diseases are heroin addicts more prone to?**	Endocarditis, pneumonia, human immunodeficiency virus (HIV), hepatitis, and cellulitis

Diagnosis

How is a heroin "high" described?	An intensely pleasurable feeling throughout the body
! **What are signs and symptoms of opiate intoxication?**	**Constricted pupils (miosis),** drowsiness, nausea, vomiting, constipation, slurred speech, hypotension, bradycardia, and **respiratory depression**
Which opiate when taken with monoamine oxidase inhibitors (MAOIs) can lead to serotonin syndrome?	Meperidine (Demerol) along with an MAOI may lead to **serotonin syndrome:** hyperthermia, rigidity, and labile blood pressure.
How long after use will opiates remain detectable in the urine and blood?	Varies by type of opiate (ie, heroin vs methadone), but generally 1-5 days
What can lead to a false positive result in a urine screen for opiates?	Recent ingestion of large quantities of poppy seeds (bagels, muffins, etc)
! **What are the three most common signs of an opiate overdose?**	Miosis, altered mental status, and respiratory depression
! **How can opiate use be determined empirically?**	If a patient with suspected opiate overdose recovers consciousness rapidly after the administration of IV naloxone (Narcan), then opiates are almost definitely the offending drug.
How is an opiate overdose treated?	With IV naloxone (Narcan)
What are common signs and symptoms of opiate withdrawal?	**Pupillary dilatation, lacrimation or rhinorrhea, piloerection or goose bumps (think "cold turkey"),** diarrhea, dysphoria, **yawning,** myalgias, nausea, vomiting, anxiety
What is the time course of opiate withdrawal?	Withdrawal symptoms from short-acting drugs such as heroin or morphine start within 8-12 hours after the last dose and reach peak severity ~48 hours after the last dose.

Is opiate withdrawal life threatening?

No. Unlike alcohol withdrawal, **opiate withdrawal is not life threatening,** but it is extremely uncomfortable.

Withdrawal from which opiate can lead to seizures?

Meperidine (Demerol)

Treatment

What is the treatment for acute opiate withdrawal symptoms?

Clonidine, a centrally acting alpha-2 receptor antagonist, decreases noradrenergic and hence sympathetic output.

Does clonidine decrease drug cravings?

No. Although it is very effective in treating the symptoms, it will not curb opiate cravings.

What medications are used to treat opiate (especially heroin) dependence?

- Methadone: low-potency, long-acting opiate receptor agonist
- Buprenorphine: long-acting, opiate receptor mixed agonist/antagonist
- Naltrexone

What advantages does buprenorphine have over methadone?

Since it is a mixed agonist/antagonist, it is safer in overdose and has less potential for abuse.

What is Suboxone?

Combination of buprenorphine and opioid antagonist naloxone used to treat opiate dependence. The addition of naloxone serves to deter users from injecting Suboxone, as injection of naloxone can cause withdrawal symptoms.

COCAINE AND AMPHETAMINES

Epidemiology and Etiology

What is the mechanism of action of cocaine?

It blocks dopamine, norepinephrine, and serotonin reuptake into the presynaptic terminal, thereby potentiating the sympathomimetic effects of these catecholamines.

Give examples of some amphetamines.	Dextroamphetamine (Dexedrine), methamphetamine (aka "crysal meth"), methylphenidate (Ritalin), 3,4-methylenedioxymethamphetamine, also known as ecstasy (MDMA)
What is the mechanism of action of most amphetamines?	They release endogenous catecholamines from nerve endings and are catecholamine receptor agonists in the central and peripheral nervous system.
What are Food and Drug Administration (FDA) approved uses of amphetamines?	Narcolepsy, extremely low energy symptoms in select patients with depression, and attention deficit hyperactivity disorder (ADHD)

Diagnosis

What are the effects of cocaine and amphetamines?	They are CNS stimulants producing euphoria, labile blood pressure, **tachycardia** or bradycardia, **pupillary dilatation, psychomotor agitation** or retardation, nausea, weight loss, chills, diaphoresis, confusion, seizures, cardiac arrhythmias, hallucinations, fever, respiratory depression, and **transient psychosis**.
! **What type of hallucination is most common after cocaine use?**	Tactile hallucinations, especially "formication," or the sensation that bugs are crawling on (or under) the skin. Formication can also be seen in alcohol withdrawal.
High doses of cocaine or amphetamines can lead to a psychosis that may be difficult to differentiate from the psychosis in what psychiatric disorder?	Schizophrenia, paranoid type
! **In patients presenting with chest pain and a history of substance abuse, what must be included in the differential diagnosis?**	Cocaine-induced myocardial infarction (MI). Cocaine is a potent vasoconstrictor and can also cause vasospasm. Excessive amounts may lead to MIs and ischemic strokes.
Urine drug tests screen for what cocaine metabolite?	Benzoylecgonine

How long after the last use of cocaine will a urine sample remain positive?
Up to 3 days, but often longer in chronic users (even up to 1 week)

How long after the last use of amphetamine will a urine sample remain positive?
1-3 days

Treatment

What is the treatment for cocaine/amphetamine addiction?
Benzodiazepines and antipsychotics can be used in the acute setting to treat agitation, but the long-term treatment should include group therapy and 12-step groups.

What are the signs and symptoms of cocaine or amphetamine withdrawal?
Depression, fatigue, headache, diaphoresis, myalgias, hunger, **constricted pupils**

What is the treatment for withdrawal?
Since the withdrawal is self-limited and not life threatening, the only treatment is supportive care.

PHENCYCLIDINE (PCP)

What is a common street name for PCP?
"Angel Dust"

What is PCPs mechanism of action?
It is an antagonist at the N-methyl-d-aspartate (NMDA) glutamate receptor and activates dopaminergic neurons.

! **What are the signs and symptoms of PCP intoxication?**
Rotatory nystagmus, ataxia, agitation, hypertension, tachycardia, hallucinations, recklessness, seizures, and coma

What sort of behavior is specifically associated with PCP intoxication?
Violent behavior is a common effect of PCP use, and patients who are suspected to have used PCP should be carefully observed as they may be a danger to themselves and to others.

How long after last use will a urine screen for PCP remain positive?
1 week

What lab abnormalities may be observed in patients who have recently used PCP?

Elevated creatinine phosphokinase (CPK) and AST

What is the treatment for PCP intoxication?

- Blood pressure normalization
- Benzodiazepines or antipsychotics for agitation and psychosis
- Diazepam for seizure treatment/prevention
- Acidification of urine with ammonium chloride and ascorbic acid to enhance renal excretion

What are the signs and symptoms of PCP withdrawal?

There generally are none.

HALLUCINOGENS

What are some examples of hallucinogens?

Lysergic acid diethylamide (LSD), mushrooms, mescaline

What are the effects of LSD?

The drug produces euphoric or dysphoric "trips" **(hallucinations and perceptual changes), pupillary dilation,** tremors, tachycardia, palpitations, and diaphoresis.

Are hallucinogens physically addicting?

No, they are not physically addicting, but they can produce psychological dependence.

What are long-term complications of LSD use?

Psychosis and recurrent visual hallucinations

What is the treatment for hallucinogen intoxication?

Reassurance and antipsychotic medications in severe cases

"CLUB DRUGS"

What is "Ecstasy"?

Ecstasy is MDMA, a drug with mixed stimulant and hallucinogenic properties that produces a euphoric effect.

What are the effects of Ecstasy?

- Subjective: alteration in consciousness, feelings of empathy/compassion toward others, euphoria, intensified perception (especially tactile), mild psychedelia
- Side effects: difficulty concentrating, lack of appetite, dry mouth, **bruxism** (grinding of teeth)
- After effects (can last 3-7 days or longer): depression, anxiety, fatigue

What are the acute risks of using Ecstasy?

Hyperthermia and hyponatremia. Continuous activity (eg, dancing) without sufficient rest or rehydration may cause body temperature to rise to dangerous levels, and loss of fluid via excessive perspiration puts the body at further risk.

Long-term use of Ecstasy may lead to loss of what type of neurons?

Fine diameter serotonergic neurons

What is "Special K"?

Ketamine; a dissociative anesthetic that has hallucinogenic effects

How will users describe an intense high from Special K?

"A near-death experience" or "K-hole"

What are other signs of Special K intoxication?

Tachycardia and tachypnea

What is "GHB"?

GHB is gamma-hydroxybutyrate and is also known as the date rape drug due to its depressant and memory loss effects.

What are complications from high doses of GHB?

Respiratory depression, coma, and death

MARIJUANA

What is the active ingredient in marijuana?

The cannabis plant produces THC or tetrahydro-cannabinol.

What are the effects of marijuana?

Euphoria, tachycardia, **paranoia,** poor concentration, **poor memory,** avolition, impaired coordination and judgment, increased appetite, and **conjunctival injection**

What properties of marijuana have been used for treatment of patients?

- Antiemetic properties used in cancer patients undergoing chemotherapy
- Appetite stimulant properties used in cancer patients
- Decreases intraocular pressure, which is useful in treatment of glaucoma
- Pain relief in chronic pain patients

What are serious complications from marijuana use?

Psychosis and delirium

What disease does early marijuana use increase risk for?

Recent research suggests that regular use of marijuana before age 15 increases risk for developing schizophrenia several-fold.

How long do urine screens for marijuana remain positive?

Daily use will result in positive screens up to 4 weeks after last use; less frequent use can result in positive screens for up to 1 week after last use.

What are the symptoms of marijuana withdrawal?

Sometimes there can be mild irritability and insomnia

What is the treatment for marijuana withdrawal?

Supportive

CAFFEINE

What is the mechanism of action of caffeine?

It increases cyclic adenosine monophosphate (cAMP) and acts via the dopaminergic system to exert a stimulant effect.

How much caffeine is in an average cup of coffee and tea?

- Coffee: 100-150 mg per cup
- Tea: 40-60 mg per cup

What are the signs and symptoms of caffeine intoxication?

Anxiety, tachycardia, insomnia, diaphoresis, GI distress, and restlessness

Ingestion of >1 and >10 g of caffeine may lead to what complications?

- >1 g: tinnitus and arrhythmias
- >10 g: seizures, respiratory failure, and death

What is the treatment for caffeine intoxication?

Supportive

What are the signs and symptoms of caffeine withdrawal?

Headache, nausea, anxiety, drowsiness, and mood lability

What is the treatment for caffeine withdrawal?

Taper caffeine intake and treatment of symptoms

NICOTINE

What is the mechanism of action of nicotine?

It stimulates nicotinic acetylcholine (ACh) receptors of both divisions of the autonomic nervous system (sympathetic and parasympathetic).

What are the signs and symptoms of nicotine intoxication?

Insomnia, restlessness, increased GI motility decreased appetite, and anxiety

! **What are the effects of cigarette smoking in pregnancy?**

Low birth weight and persistent pulmonary hypertension of the newborn (PPHN)

What are the signs and symptoms of nicotine withdrawal?

Anxiety, increased appetite, irritability, insomnia, and cigarette (nicotine) craving

What are the different therapeutic approaches to smoking cessation?

- Counseling.
- Nicotine replacement with gum, nasal spray (provides the fastest method of nicotine delivery of all nicotine replacement products), inhaler, or skin patch.
- Bupropion (Zyban)—an antidepressant that is FDA approved for smoking cessation.
- Varenicline (Chantix)—agonist of and blocks certain nicotinic ACh receptors. Initial research suggests that it is more effective than bupropion (Zyban) for smoking cessation.
- Clonidine.

How does Zyban differ from Wellbutrin?

They are identical: simply different trade names for bupropion based on their different uses.

CLINICAL VIGNETTES

A 21-year-old woman is brought to the emergency room (ER) after her friends found her passed out in an acquaintance's dorm room. Her friends say that they "were all out partying and met some boys at a bar," after which they went back to their dorms for more drinks. The patient apparently went off into one of the boys' rooms but she does not remember anything after leaving her friends. On examination, there are signs of vaginal trauma suggestive of rape but the patient cannot recall having intercourse. What drug may she have unknowingly ingested?

GHB; gamma-hydroxybutyrate (GHB), also known as the "date rape drug," has profound depressive and memory loss effects. A serum GHB screen should be performed in this patient as well as a rape screen.

An 18-year-old woman is brought into the ER by her mother who reports having found the girl on the bathroom floor confused and drowsy. According to the mother, the only medication that her daughter takes is alprazolam (Xanax) for anxiety. In addition, the mother reports that her daughter has never had a seizure, but her 12-year-old brother did have seizures as a younger child. Her vitals are: T 98.7°F, HR 66, BP 118/76 mm Hg, RR 6, O2 saturation 98% on room air. The patient is arousable to painful stimuli and her pupils are reactive. What is the proper management of this patient?

Airway management ± flumazenil; airway protection is the chief concern and intubation may be necessary in patients with compromised respiratory drive or function. Although benzodiazepines do not generally cause respiratory depression that is as severe as that resulting from barbiturates, clinicians must still be alert to respiratory status in benzodiazepine overdose. A toxicology screen should be performed, and flumazenil should be considered to reverse the effects if the screen is positive for benzodiazepines (such as alprazolam). However, flumazenil can lower seizure threshold, and given the patient's family history, care should be taken if it must be administered. Activated charcoal via a nasogastric tube can also be considered to halt the gastrointestinal (GI) absorption of any remaining pills in the patient's stomach.

A 45-year-old man is admitted to the ICU after a car accident. He has three fractured ribs and a few minor contusions, but no neurologic deficits. His vitals are T 101.2°F, HR 104, BP 126/75, RR 20, O2 saturation 99%. On examination, his pupils are 4 mm and reactive bilaterally. His patellar and biceps reflexes are 3+ bilaterally. His toxicity screen from admissions shows a blood alcohol level (BAL) of 30 mg/dL. What is the proper management of this patient?

Airway management and withdrawal prevention; airway protection is always the paramount concern. With his documented history of alcohol use and signs/symptoms of sympathetic hyperactivity (fever, tachycardia, and hyperreflexia), this patient is at risk for alcohol withdrawal. Although he may not require intubation now, threshold for intubation should be low in patients withdrawing from alcohol. His BAL is relatively low, and given the history, this likely means that he has nearly finished metabolizing the alcohol in his system. It is at this time that patients are at greatest risk for withdrawal and delirium tremens (DTs). It is important to note that a patient's BAL does not need to be very high nor zero for them to begin withdrawing. Another major concern is that this patient will begin to seize and/or go into DTs, as occurrence of these problems is most common within the first 48 hours after his last drink. Therefore, the patient should be started on a lorazepam drip and slowly tapered over the next few days.

A 37-year-old homeless man is brought into the ED after being picked up by the emergency medical technicians (EMTs) in front of an outdoor café. Apparently the man was yelling at the customers seated at tables about nonsensical things. He kept asking them why he was at the zoo. On examination, he was disheveled, malodorous, and confused. He had trouble keeping his balance and walking a straight line. On extraocular muscle examination, the physician asked him to follow a finger out to his right side with his eyes while keeping his head straight ahead. His left eye moved medially to his nose while his right eye could not move laterally to the finger. BAL was elevated. What is the treatment for this disease process?

Wernicke encephalopathy, treat with immediate intravenous thiamine infusion; prolonged alcohol abuse leads to thiamine deficiency. Because the mamillary bodies and dorsomedial nucleus of the thalamus are dependent on thiamine, its deficiency may result in Wernicke-Korsakoff syndrome. This patient demonstrates the classical triad of ataxia, abnormal eye movements including nystagmus and lateral gaze palsy, and confusion.

A man comes to the ER with no identification and clearly smelling of alcohol. He begins to tell an elaborate story about how he was tossed out of his car near the ER. When you return to the room 30 minutes later, he forgets that he has ever met you. On examination, you observe a jaundiced middle-aged man, with small testes and enlarged breasts. His temperature is 98.0°F, HR is 86, and BP is 134/86. What syndrome do you believe this man may have and how can he be managed?

Korsakoff syndrome; the patient is showing physical signs of advanced alcoholism (jaundice, testicular atrophy, gynecomastia). He is also confabulating and exhibiting anterograde amnesia, both of which are signs of Korsakoff syndrome. Two-thirds of Korsakoff cases are irreversible but thiamine and folate should be supplemented.

A 27-year-old law student comes to her primary care physician complaining of a rapid heart beat, abdominal pain, diarrhea, and lightheadedness almost every morning over the past week. These symptoms tend to lessen in severity during the course of the day, but are very troublesome to her. She recognizes that exams are "stressing her out," but she says that tests never worried her before. Before making the diagnosis of panic attacks or panic disorder, what habits should the physician inquire about?

Caffeine intake and cigarette smoking (in addition to other drug use); these substances can contribute significantly to anxiety and its systemic symptoms. Their use should be limited if panic disorder is a suspected diagnosis.

An 18-year-old woman is admitted to the ER after she attacks her roommate in a frenzy. On questioning, she states that she knows that her roommate has been "following her" and "tape recording her conversations." She appears alert and oriented but goes off on long tangents before answering the doctor's questions. She admits to "partying all night long." The woman then abruptly terminates the interview, refusing to answer any more questions and claiming that she "can't trust anyone." According to her roommate, she has no history of such behavior. A urine toxicology screen comes back positive. What is the likely diagnosis and causative agent?

Substance-induced psychotic disorder, which is defined by the onset of psychotic symptoms within 1 month of use of/withdrawal from agent. Cocaine, amphetamine, PCP, and ketamine can all produce psychotic symptoms in the acute stage.

A 39-year-old homeless man is found in an alley by police. He is mumbling and is having difficulty walking. As you examine him in the ER, you notice that his palms and cheeks are red. You also can smell alcohol on his breath. As you attempt to interview the patient, he becomes unresponsive. What should be your first intervention at this point?

Protect the patient's airway; the clinical picture in this case is common for alcoholic patients. The rosy cheeks and palms are additional signs of chronic alcohol use. In a semiconscious or unconscious alcoholic patient, intubation (with or without sedation) should be considered. Alcoholics tend to aspirate if they vomit and therefore airway protection is key to prevent further complications.

The patient in the previous vignette is intubated. The nurse is about to start IV D5½ NS fluids. What is your concern with this routine therapy?

Wernicke-Korsakoff syndrome; if the patient is started on these fluids prior to thiamine supplementation, the glucose will further deplete his thiamine stores. Therefore, the patient should receive thiamine first and the necessary IV fluids after. Thiamine replenishment should prevent Wernicke-Korsakoff syndrome in most malnourished alcoholic patients.

A 45-year-old man has begun to drink heavily every night following the tragic death of his wife a year ago. He is consistently late for work and progressively spends more time alone. He tries to stop drinking but gets the "shakes" and then drinks more. He is spending more and more money each month to buy alcohol because he now needs a pint of vodka to get as drunk as he once got from a few shots. Would this be classified as alcohol abuse or alcohol dependence?

Alcohol dependence; this is an example of alcohol dependence, as the man exhibits signs of tolerance (requiring more alcohol to achieve same desired effect), withdrawal ("the shakes"), and has a desire to cut down on his alcohol consumption. Since he has exhibited these three characteristics in the past 12 months, he fits the *DSM-IV* (*Diagnostic and Statistical Manual of Mental Disorders, Fourth Edition*) classification of alcohol dependence. Note that tolerance and withdrawal are not necessary per se for a diagnosis of substance dependence; rather, a person must meet any three of the seven *DSM* criteria for dependence.

A 54-year-old man is brought to the hospital by the police after causing trouble at home. The man works as a wood carver. He was in the Navy for 25 years until he was dishonorably discharged because of continued alcohol abuse. Over the last 4 years, he has been living with his elderly parents who refuse to deal with his alcohol problem any longer. The parents report that their son cannot hold a job, rarely sells a piece of his wood carving, and makes a mess at home. When questioning the man, he is slightly confused and perseverates about his skill as a wood carver. He is able to recount the earlier years of his Navy career, but is unable to account for the happenings of the last 7 years. He cannot exactly remember when or why he left the Navy. On memory testing, he is able to repeat three words immediately after the physician says them; however, he can remember only one of the words after 3 minutes and none of the words after 5 minutes. He is unaware of current political, local, or world events. What is the most likely diagnosis?

Korsakoff psychosis; alcohol abuse is a leading cause of substance-related amnestic disorder. Korsakoff psychosis (alcohol-induced persistent amnestic disorder) can persist after proper treatment of Wernicke encephalopathy with thiamine infusion. The diagnosis of Korsakoff psychosis is appropriate in this patient because of his long-standing alcohol abuse history, impaired short-term memory, and permanent gap in memory of a definitive period in time due to anterograde amnesia. Damage to the mamillary bodies causes the amnestic symptoms seen in Wernicke-Korsakoff syndrome.

Paramedics bring a young, unidentified man into the ER. He was found asleep on a park bench and was difficult to arouse. His HR is 45 and BP is 106/70. On examination, he is diaphoretic and unable to answer questions. His pupils are 1 mm and minimally reactive bilaterally. As the nurse attempts to draw blood from his forearm, you notice multiple track marks. Before the blood work results are finished, what drug can be given to help reverse his state?

Naloxone (Narcan); the history is suggestive of heroin overdose, and the pinpoint pupils are pathognomonic in this situation for opiate intoxication. Naloxone (Narcan) can be given to patients with suspected heroin overdose to act as an opiate antagonist and reverse the heroin's effect. Most patients will recover to some degree within seconds or minutes of Narcan administration.

A 26-year-old man walks into the urgent care clinic. You attempt to interview the man but cannot get a word in as he speaks extremely quickly about animals crawling all over him. He keeps scratching his skin but you cannot observe any skin abnormalities aside from the obvious scratch marks. He is difficult to interview because he will not stop talking. His vitals are: T 98.6°F, HR 96, BP 135/80, RR 18, O2 saturation 100% on room air. You suspect intoxication of some sort and perform a urine drug screen. What metabolite would you expect to see in the urine?

Benzoylecgonine; it is likely that this man used cocaine recently as he appears to be having tactile hallucinations ("cocaine bugs") and is clearly in a "stimulated" state. Benzoylecgonine, a cocaine metabolite, will usually remain in the urine for up to 3 days (and possibly up to 1 week).

A 19-year-old man is brought into the ER accompanied by three police officers. He is kicking at everything in sight and needs to be restrained to the bed. He will not calm down and needs to be sedated with Haldol. The police tell you that he is being held as a suspect in a violent assault and battery. What drug did the patient most likely take and what physical sign is virtually pathognomonic for intoxication with this drug?

Phencyclidine (PCP); PCP (aka "angel dust") produces hallucinations and is often linked to violent behavior. Rotatory nystagmus is pathognomonic for PCP intoxication.

A 23-year-old man is brought to the ER by friends who are concerned because "he's acting really weird...like almost too friendly and hyper." On exam the patient appears flushed, diaphoretic, and distracted. His pupils are dilated. You notice that he seems anxious and that his jaw is clenched. His labs come back and his sodium level is borderline low. What drug did the patient most likely take?

Ecstasy (MDMA), a drug with mixed stimulant and hallucinogenic properties. Typical effects of Ecstasy are feelings of empathy/compassion toward others, euphoria, and mild psychedelia. Physical signs include dilated pupils, diaphoresis, flushing, and bruxism (grinding of teeth). Acute risks include hyperthermia and hyponatremia due to continuous activity (eg, dancing) without sufficient rest or rehydration. There is some evidence that long-term use of Ecstasy results in damage to fine diameter serotonergic neurons.

CHAPTER 11

Eating Disorders

INTRODUCTION

What are eating disorders?

A group of conditions characterized by abnormal eating habits that may involve either insufficient or excessive food intake to the detriment of an individual's physical and emotional health

What are examples of harmful eating habits?

- Abnormal regulation of food intake—restricted food intake or episodes of binge eating
- Abnormal diet—restricted range of foods
- Purging—evacuation of food through vomiting or taking laxatives, diuretics, or enemas, or engaging in intense exercise

How common are "weight concerns" in contemporary US society?

According to the 2003 Youth Risk Behavior Survey, 36% of adolescent girls believed that they were overweight, and 59% were attempting to lose weight.

What are examples of abnormal thinking seen in patients with eating disorders?

Dichotomous (all-or-none) thinking, decreased concentration, disturbed body image, disturbed perception (eg, denial of fatigue, weakness, or hunger), a sense of ineffectiveness and associated preoccupation with control

ANOREXIA NERVOSA

Epidemiology and Etiology

What is the lifetime prevalence of anorexia nervosa?	0.3%-1%
What is the prevalence of anorexia nervosa among young adults?	Up to 4%
How has the incidence of anorexia nervosa changed over the past 10 years?	It has increased tenfold.
Are men and women equally affected?	No. It is 10-20 times more common in women than men.
What is the typical age of onset of anorexia nervosa?	Mean age of 17, with a range from 10 to 30
Where is anorexia nervosa most common?	In developed countries, higher socioeconomic classes, and professions requiring a thin physique (eg, ballet)
! **What is the mortality rate for anorexia nervosa?**	10%-20% over 10-30 years
What are the most common causes of death in anorexia nervosa?	Severe and chronic starvation, sudden death due to cardiac failure, and suicide
! **What other psychiatric disorders have a high rate of concurrence with anorexia nervosa?**	Major depression and obsessive-compulsive disorder

Diagnosis

! **What are the *DSM-IV* (*Diagnostic and Statistical Manual of Mental Disorders, Fourth Edition*) diagnostic criteria for anorexia nervosa?**

- Refusal to maintain at least 85% of ideal body weight
- Intense fear of gaining weight or becoming fat
- Disturbed body image
- **Amenorrhea** in postmenarchal women

! What are the subtypes of anorexia nervosa?

- Restrictive—controls weight through food restriction and exercise; associated with **obsessive-compulsive traits** such as inflexibility, limited spontaneity, and concern with control
- Binge eating/purging type—controls weight through binging and purging; associated with depression and substance abuse

What is the differential diagnosis of anorexia nervosa?

Medical condition causing weight loss (eg, cancer), major depression, bulimia, and other psychiatric disorders (eg, obsessive-compulsive disorder and body dysmorphic disorder)

! What physical findings are associated with eating disorders?

- Signs of malnutrition
  - Emaciation
  - Hypotension
  - Bradycardia
  - **Lanugo (ie, fine hair on trunk)**
  - Peripheral edema
- Signs of purging
  - **Eroded dental enamel (caused by emesis)**
  - **Scarred/scratched hands (or "Russell's sign," from inducing emesis with fingers)**
  - Parotid gland hypertrophy
  - Esophageal/gastric tears (from vomiting)

! What laboratory findings are associated with eating disorders?

- Signs of malnutrition
  - Normochromic, normocytic anemia
  - Elevated liver enzymes
  - Abnormal electrolytes
  - Hypercholesterolemia
  - Low estrogen and testosterone
  - Abnormal neuroendocrine responses
  - Bradycardia
  - Reduced brain mass
  - Cardiac arrhythmias (eg, prolonged QT interval and ventricular tachycardia)
- Signs of purging
  - Emesis: metabolic alkalosis, hypochloremia, hypokalemia
  - Laxative abuse: metabolic acidosis

What neurotransmitter and peptide abnormalities are seen in anorexia nervosa?	Decreased norepinephrine; increased serotonin, corticotrophin-releasing factor (CRF), neuropeptide Y, and cholecystokinin (CCK)
What is the effect of serotonin on eating behaviors?	It is thought to promote satiety.
What skeletal disease can occur as a complication of anorexia nervosa?	Osteoporosis
What gastrointestinal abnormalities are seen in anorexic patients?	Diminished motility delayed gastric emptying, bloating, constipation, acute gastric dilation or gastric rupture, and abdominal pain
What is the typical course of anorexia nervosa?	Variable—patients can completely recover, have fluctuating symptoms with relapses, or progressively deteriorate.
! **What factors are associated with a worse outcome?**	Longer duration of illness, older age of onset, prior psychiatric admission, poor childhood social adjustment, premorbid personality difficulties, and disturbed familial relationships

Treatment

What is the first step in the treatment of anorexic patients?	Obtain their cooperation in the treatment program
What are the goals in treating anorexia nervosa?	Correct metabolic disturbances, restore a safe weight and normal eating behaviors, and improve the accuracy of individual's body image.
! **What are the indications for hospitalization in a patient with an eating disorder?**	Substantial weight loss (ie, person is more than 20% below ideal body weight), inability to gain weight during outpatient treatment, metabolic crises, and suicidal crises
What modalities are used to treat anorexia nervosa?	Psychotherapy (eg, behavioral and family therapy), supervised weight gain programs, and medications

What is the most effective form of behavioral therapy for anorexia nervosa?

Operant conditioning—positive reinforcement for healthy behaviors; negative reinforcement for unhealthy behaviors

Describe the medications used in the treatment of anorexia nervosa.

- Cyproheptadine—5-HT antagonist that facilitates weight gain
- Tricyclic antidepressants (TCAs) and selective serotonin reuptake inhibitors (SSRIs)—treat comorbid depression

At what rate should weight gain occur for anorexic patients during a refeeding treatment?

1-2 kg/week or 0.25 lb/day

What complications can result from refeeding a patient too quickly?

Acute gastric dilation, congestive heart failure, and pancreatitis

What is a good way to assess anorexic patients' risk for fractures secondary to osteoporosis?

Bone mineral densitometry

BULIMIA NERVOSA

Epidemiology and Etiology

What is the prevalence of bulimia nervosa among adolescent females?

1%-3%

Are men and women equally affected by bulimia nervosa?

No. It is nine times more common in women.

What percentage of patients with anorexia nervosa develop binging/purging symptoms?

Up to 50%

What is the typical age of onset of bulimia nervosa?

Mean age of 18, with a range of 12-35

What Axis I disorders have a high rate of concurrence with bulimia nervosa?

Mood disorders, substance abuse, impulse control disorders, and anxiety disorders

What is the etiology of bulimia nervosa?

The following factors have been implicated:

- Psychological—issues about guilt, helplessness, self-control, and body image
- Biologic—based on frequent association with mood disorders

Diagnosis

! **What are the *DSM-IV* diagnostic criteria for bulimia nervosa?**

- Recurrent episodes of binge eating
- Recurrent, inappropriate compensatory behavior—self-induced vomiting; misuse of laxatives, diuretics, enemas, or other medications; fasting; or excessive exercise
- Binge eating and compensatory behaviors occur at least twice a week for 3 months
- Perception of self-worth is unduly influenced by body shape and weight

What compensatory behavior is most often used by individuals with bulimia nervosa?

80%-90% of bulimic patients engage in **self-induced vomiting**.

What are the subtypes of bulimia nervosa?

- *Purging*—involves vomiting, laxatives, diuretics, enemas, or other medications
- *Nonpurging*—involves excessive exercise or fasting

! **What distinguishes patients with bulimia from those with anorexia?**

- Bulimic patients typically maintain a **normal weight** and may even be overweight.
- Bulimic patients tend to be **more embarrassed by and** secretive about their symptoms.
- Bulimic patients' symptoms are "**ego-dystonic,**" or distressing, so they may be more likely to seek help.

What is the differential diagnosis of bulimia nervosa?

Anorexia nervosa, binge eating/purging type; major depressive disorder with atypical features and borderline personality disorder

! **What personality type may be associated with bulimia nervosa?**

Borderline personality type is seen in up to 50% of patients with bulimia.

What physical findings are associated with bulimia nervosa?

See signs of purging

What laboratory findings are associated with bulimia nervosa?

See signs of purging

! **What changes occur in amylase levels with bulimia nervosa?**

Elevation in salivary subtype of amylase

What is "Russell's sign"?

Presence of scarring on the knuckles secondary to repeated self-induction of emesis

What substance is sometimes ingested by patients with eating disorders to induce vomiting?

Ipecac

What are the signs and symptoms of ipecac toxicity?

Precordial pain, dyspnea, and generalized muscle weakness associated with hypotension, tachycardia, abnormalities in the electroencephalography (EEG), elevated liver enzymes, and elevated erythrocyte sedimentation rate

What medical complications can develop from ipecac ingestion?

Cardiomyopathy and toxic myopathy

What is the typical course of bulimia nervosa?

50% recover fully with treatment; 50% have a chronic course with fluctuating symptoms.

How does the prognosis for bulimia compare to anorexia nervosa?

Bulimia has a better prognosis.

Treatment

What are the treatment goals of bulimia nervosa?

Restore healthy eating behaviors, improve the individual's self-image, and reduce the associated mood and personality symptoms

! Describe the treatment modalities used in bulimia nervosa.

- Cognitive-behavioral therapy—focuses on altering distorted body image and rigid rules regarding food consumption and dieting, and recognition of events that trigger episodes of binge eating
- Antidepressant medications—SSRIs (first-line), TCAs, monoamine oxidase inhibitors (MAOIs)
- Psychodynamic psychotherapy—useful for those patients with comorbid borderline personality disorder

What is a good way to assess reduction of vomiting in patients who deny purging episodes?

Serum amylase level. It will be elevated in patients who binge and vomit.

What is the response-prevention technique?

Binging and purging patients are required to stay in an observed area for 2-3 hours after every meal to prevent purging.

BINGE EATING DISORDER

What factors contribute to the current obesity epidemic in the United States?

Genetic factors, overeating, and lack of activity have all been implicated.

What is the prevalence of binge eating disorder?

0.7%-4%

What is the usual age of onset of binge eating?

Late adolescence or early 20s, often coming soon after significant weight loss from dieting

What percentage of obese individuals seeking weight-loss treatment have binge eating disorder?

A mean of 30%; ranges from 15% to 50%

Are men and women equally affected by binge eating disorder?

No. It is 1.5 times more common in women.

What are the *DSM-IV* diagnostic criteria for binge eating disorder?

- Recurrent episodes of binge eating
- Severe distress over binge eating
- Bingeing occurs at least 2 days a week for 6 months and is not associated with compensatory behaviors
- Three or more of the following are present:
- Eating very rapidly
- Eating until uncomfortably full
- Eating large amounts when not hungry
- Eating alone due to embarrassment over eating habits
- Feeling disgusted, depressed, or guilty after overeating

Binge eating disorder is listed in the *DSM-IV* category of Eating Disorder NOS (not otherwise specified).

What is the treatment for binge eating disorder?

- Individual psychotherapy and behavioral therapy
- Strict diet and exercise program
- Comorbid psychiatric disorders treated as necessary

CLINICAL VIGNETTES

A 16-year-old girl is brought to her family physician by her mother, who is distraught about her daughter's recent rapid weight loss. Her current height and weight are 5′4″ and 88 lb, respectively. Her mother claims that she refuses to eat and spends long hours jogging at a nearby park. What is the next appropriate step in management?

Hospitalization for anorexia; the physician should hospitalize her, as she is more than 20% below her ideal weight. The most important treatment goals should be to correct the physiologic effects of her starvation and restore her to a safe weight.

A 22-year-old man reports to his primary care physician for an annual checkup. His vital signs are T 98.5°F, HR 76, BP 115/80, and RR 20. His body mass index (BMI) is 31. When questioned about his lifestyle, the man admits to not exercising much and "occasionally" overeating. When pressed for more details, the man describes eating large amounts of food a few times a week, after which he will often have feelings of physical discomfort and guilt. He is interested in weight loss programs. What is the diagnosis and appropriate treatment?

Binge eating disorder; treat with psychotherapy, behavioral therapy, and diet/exercise. The man exhibits the typical symptoms of binge eating disorder, including frequent, recurrent episodes of binge eating, as well as physical and emotional distress over binge eating. Treatment includes individual psychotherapy and behavioral therapy and strict diet and exercise programs.

A 21-year-old, emaciated woman is seen in the ER for "malnutrition." Physical examination is unremarkable aside from the presence of fine, thin hair on the trunk of her body. Laboratory results are as follows: Na 140, K 3, Cl 97, HCO3 18, and pH 7.29. Her BMI is 17. What is the likely diagnosis and cause of her abnormal lab findings?

Anorexia nervosa, purging type; her abnormally low BMI suggests the diagnosis of anorexia, as bulimic patients typically maintain normal body weight. This woman also has a metabolic acidosis, as indicated by her low bicarbonate and pH levels. The likely cause of this acid-base disorder is diarrhea secondary to laxative abuse. The fine hair on the trunk of her body is lanugo, which is a physical sign of malnutrition.

A 15-year-old girl is brought to her physician for being significantly underweight. On questioning, she expresses dissatisfaction with her body and wishes that she was "a few pounds lighter." Her last menstrual period was 1 year ago. She complains of a loss of interest in her hobbies and spends most of the day in bed. For the past month, she has been unable to concentrate on her schoolwork, and she is now in danger of failing some of her classes. What is her diagnosis? How should she be treated?

Anorexia nervosa and major depression. Treat with psychotherapy, weight gain programs, and antidepressants; major depression and obsessive-compulsive disorder are the psychiatric disorders most often seen in patients with anorexia. Psychotherapy (eg, behavioral [with a focus on operant conditioning] therapy and family therapy) and supervised weight gain programs are most effective in treating anorexia nervosa. Fluoxetine and other SSRIs are useful for comorbid depression.

A 32-year-old emaciated woman with a history of anorexia is admitted to the hospital after collapsing at her workplace. According to coworkers, she has eaten very little in the past week and was appearing more and more tired. After physically examining her and obtaining labs, ER physicians determine that she is severely malnourished and start her on IV fluids so as to resuscitate her. On regaining consciousness, the patient pulls the IV out of her arm and demands to leave. The attending physician advises her that because of her condition, she should stay in the hospital for a few days so that she can be fed properly, as her malnourishment is life threatening. The patient refuses. Would it be justifiable for the ER physician to admit her to the hospital involuntarily?

Yes; since there is strong evidence that the patient is at high risk for harming herself through willful malnourishment, the ER physician would be justified in both admitting and treating the patient against her wishes.

A 19-year-old woman was recently hospitalized for being severely underweight. Since this time, she insists that she has been "eating regularly" and wishes to be discharged. She promises to continue her healthy eating behaviors on being released from the hospital. Is this sufficient for allowing her to be released?

No. The woman must maintain an agreed-upon weight; weight maintenance is the primary goal in the treatment of anorexia nervosa and supersedes all other issues; in this sense, it is not sufficient for the woman to promise to adhere to a healthy diet.

A 26-year-old woman is seen by her primary care physician for a routine checkup. She is 5′3″ and 110 lb (BMI 19.5). On physical examination, the physician palpates a hypertrophic parotid gland. The rest of the examination is normal except for some scarring on the dorsal aspect of the woman's right hand. On questioning as to the cause of this scarring, the woman becomes quite embarrassed and claims that she does not know the reason. The physician attempts to discuss the woman's eating habits, but the woman is quite evasive, saying only that she feels a lot of pressure "to stay thin." What is the likely diagnosis and subsequent treatment? What is this patient's prognosis?

Bulimia nervosa; treat with cognitive-behavioral therapy, antidepressants, and psychodynamic psychotherapy. Fifty percent recovery rate; a hyper-trophic parotid gland and scarring of the hands are both physical signs of repeated self-induced emesis, which is the most frequently seen compensatory behavior in bulimic patients. Treatment for bulimia includes cognitive-behavioral therapy, anti-depressant medications (SSRIs are first-line treatment), and psychodynamic psychotherapy, which can be useful for those patients with concurrent borderline personality disorder. Prognosis for bulimia is better than anorexia: 50% of patients completely recover.

What laboratory finding is typically abnormal in the patient in the previous vignette and how can it be used to assess treatment?

The salivary component of serum amylase will be elevated in patients who binge and vomit. It should decrease following cessation of this behavior.

A 17-year-old girl is referred to a psychiatrist for evaluation following a period of dramatic weight loss. Her mother claims that she has lost "nearly 20 pounds" in a 6-month period. She is currently 5'5" and 100 lb. On questioning, the girl states that she "prefers to eat less food" in order to lose some of her "excess fat." She also wishes she was "a little skinnier." What is the likely diagnosis? What additional finding would confirm this diagnosis?

Anorexia nervosa. Amenorrhea would confirm the diagnosis; the patient exhibits the other symptoms of anorexia, including failure to maintain at least 85% of ideal body weight, disturbed body image, and fear of becoming fat.

An 18-year-old woman is known by her friends as an "avid exerciser." She prides herself on her ability to lose weight and is known to spend hours in front of her bedroom mirror analyzing her appearance. Despite her slight physique, she was recently overheard saying that would like to be "a lot thinner." What neurotransmitter and peptide abnormalities are thought to characterize her condition?

Decreased norepinephrine, and increased serotonin, corticotropin-releasing factor (CRF), neuropeptide Y, and cholecystokinin (CCK) are seen in anorexia nervosa.

A 23-year-old woman is brought to her primary care physician by her boyfriend, who is concerned about her health. He states that recently she has refused to eat meals with him and that he rarely sees her eat anything. The woman seems embarrassed to discuss her eating habits, and merely states that she is "not underweight." On physical examination, the physician notes that the woman has small callouses on her knuckles. He also observes that the woman appears to have poor dental hygiene. What is the likely diagnosis?

Bulimia nervosa; bulimic patients are often embarrassed of or secretive about their eating habits, and their normal weight and the presence of menstruation distinguishes them from patients with anorexia. This patient's callouses and poor dental hygiene are consistent with repeated self-induced emesis, the most frequent compensatory behavior observed in bulimic patients.

CHAPTER 12

Miscellaneous Disorders

SEXUAL DISORDERS

Sexual Dysfunction

What are sexual dysfunctions?

Disorders in the normal sexual response cycle not caused by medications or a medical condition

! **Describe sexual changes associated with aging in men.**

No change in desire; however, achievement of orgasm requires more genital contact and time, orgasm is less intense, and refractory period is increased.

Describe sexual changes associated with aging in women.

Vaginal dryness and thinning after menopause secondary to decreased estrogen

What are the disorders of sexual desire?

- *Hypoactive sexual desire disorder*: absence or decrease in desire to participate in sexual activities
- *Sexual aversion disorder*: aversion to genital sexual contact

What is a possible treatment for hypoactive sexual desire disorder in men and women?

Testosterone supplements if the patient's baseline levels are low

What are the sexual arousal disorders?

- *Female sexual arousal disorder*: inability to maintain sufficient vaginal lubrication
- *Male erectile disorder*: inability to attain an erection

What are treatments for male erectile disorder?

Medications such as yohimbine (Yocon) and sildenafil (Viagra), vacuum pumps, constrictive rings, self-injections of alprostadil (Caverject), and prosthetic implantation

! **In men who are able to masturbate and who achieve erections during sleep but are unable to achieve an erection for sex, what is the likely etiology of the erectile dysfunction?**

Psychological

What are the disorders of orgasm?

- *Female orgasmic disorder*: delayed or absent orgasm after a normal excitement phase
- *Male orgasmic disorder*: same as above
- *Premature ejaculation*: orgasm and ejaculation occur earlier than desired

What are the different treatment strategies for premature ejaculation?

- *Squeeze technique*: Man or partner squeezes the glans of his penis just prior to ejaculation in order to delay it.
- *Start-and-stop technique*: Cessation of penile contact when man is near ejaculation and resuming contact once he has become more relaxed.
- *Pharmacotherapy*: Selective serotonin reuptake inhibitors (SSRIs) may have some benefit.

What are the sexual pain disorders?

- *Dyspareunia*: genital pain with sexual intercourse
- *Vaginismus*: involuntary muscular contraction of the outer one-third of the vagina during penetration

Paraphilias

! **Define paraphilia.**

Paraphilias are sexual activities that are culturally unusual. According to the *DSM-IV* (*Diagnostic and Statistical Manual of Mental Disorders, Fourth Edition*), to be diagnosed with a paraphilia one must engage in one of these activities for at least 6 months and it must cause impairment in daily activities.

Is there a gender predominance in patients diagnosed with paraphilias?	Yes, there is a large male predominance.
What is pedophilia?	Sexual excitement derived from fantasy or engagement in sexual behavior with prepubescent children
What is exhibitionism?	Sexual excitement from exposing one's genitals to strangers
What is voyeurism?	Sexual excitement from observation of unsuspecting naked individuals
What is frotteurism?	Sexual excitement from rubbing one's genitals on unsuspecting people, usually in a crowded place (eg, in a subway)
What is fetishism?	Nonliving objects are the centerpiece of sexual fantasies or behavior (eg, shoes)
What is sexual masochism?	Sexual excitement from being the recipient of pain, embarrassment, or bondage
What is sexual sadism?	Sexual excitement from harming or inflicting pain on another
What is transvestic-fetishism?	Sexual gratification or excitement in heterosexual men wearing women's clothing
What is paraphilia not otherwise specified (NOS)?	Paraphilias not listed above, including necrophilia
What are poor prognostic factors in paraphilias?	Early age at onset, substance abuse, high frequency of paraphiliac behavior, and more than one paraphilia
What are favorable prognostic factors?	Self-referral for treatment, sense of guilt regarding paraphiliac behavior, and history of normal sexual behavior
What is the treatment for paraphilias?	The treatment is not specialized but insight-oriented psychotherapy, behavior therapy, and pharmacologic treatments have been successful.

Gender Identity Disorder

What is gender identity disorder?	A conflict between a person's actual physical gender and the one they actually identify him or herself as. For example, a person identified as a boy may actually feel and act like a girl. [NB: *DSM's* inclusion of this concept as a "disorder" is controversial, as many or most transgender people do not regard their own cross-gender feelings and behaviors as a disorder. People within the transgender community often question what a "normal" gender identity or "normal" gender role is supposed to be.]
Can people with ambiguous genitalia be diagnosed with gender identity disorder?	No
By about what age is one's gender identity typically apparent (one's internal feeling of what gender they belong to)?	Age 3

Dissociative Disorders

What are the dissociative disorders?	Disturbances of the integration of memory or identity
! Differentiate the causes of dissociative and amnestic disorders.	Amnestic disorders can be caused by medical conditions, whereas dissociative disorders occur secondary to stressful life events.
What is the most common dissociative disorder?	Dissociative amnesia

Dissociative Amnesia

What is dissociative amnesia?	Temporary inability to recall important personal information
Does dissociative amnesia affect more men or women?	Women

! According to the *DSM-IV,* how is dissociative amnesia diagnosed?

- At least one episode of inability to recall personal information usually pertaining to a stressful event.
- The amnesia cannot be attributed to simple forgetfulness or to another medical cause or by medications.
- Symptoms cause distress and impair daily functioning.

What is the typical course of dissociative amnesia?

Most patients return to baseline within days, sometimes within minutes.

What is the treatment?

The goal of treatment should be assisting patients in retrieving lost memories through psychotherapy with the assistance of lorazepam, sodium amytal, or hypnosis to help patients relax.

Dissociative Fugue

What is a dissociative fugue?

Sudden, unexplained travel, far from one's home, in combination with an inability to recall one's identity. Patients generally assume a new identity when they reach their destination and are unaware that they left their home.

What are predisposing factors?

Traumatic life events, head trauma, alcohol abuse, major depression, and epilepsy

! According to the *DSM-IV,* how is a dissociative fugue diagnosed?

- Sudden, unexpected travel accompanied by an inability to recall one's past
- Assumption of a new identity or confusion about one's identity
- Symptoms result in impairment in daily functioning
- Not attributable to other medical or pharmacologic causes

What is the typical course of a dissociative fugue?

It can last anywhere from hours to days. When the episode ends, patients reassume their true identity and are unaware of the preceding episode.

What is the treatment?

Same as dissociative amnesia

Dissociative Identity Disorder

What is the colloquial term for dissociative identity disorder?
"Multiple personality disorder"

What is dissociative identity disorder?
Disorder in which patients manifest sense of self into two or more distinct personalities

What are predisposing factors?
Female gender, childhood trauma, bipolar disorder, personality disorder, and substance abuse

What is the average age at diagnosis?
30

What is the incidence of dissociative identity disorder?
Estimates are variable, ranging from 0.015% to 14%. Although diagnoses of dissociative identity disorder seem to be increasing, many clinicians dispute its validity and believe that it is an iatrogenic condition over-diagnosed in highly suggestible individuals.

! **According to the *DSM-IV*, how is dissociative identity disorder diagnosed?**
- Presence of at least two distinct identities that are capable of controlling the patient's behavior
- Inability to recall the personal information from other personalities when one is dominant
- Not attributable to medical or pharmacologic causes

What is the typical course of the disease?
It is chronic and has a worse prognosis than other dissociative disorders.

What are treatments for dissociative personality disorder?
Treatments are controversial, but hypnosis, psychotherapy, and pharmacotherapy have all been used.

Depersonalization Disorder

What is depersonalization disorder?
A sense of being detached from one's own body, similar to recurrent "out of body" experiences

What is the most common demographic affected by this?
Women between 15 and 30 and those suffering from intense stress

What type of epilepsy can be associated with depersonalization?	Temporal lobe epilepsy
! According to the *DSM-IV*, how is depersonalization disorder diagnosed?	• Recurrent feelings of being detached from one's body • Reality testing remains normal throughout the episodes • Results in social impairment (including anxiety and depression) • Cannot be attributed to medical or pharmacologic causes
What is the typical course of depersonalization disorder?	Chronic
Can any patient describing a single out-of-body experience be diagnosed with depersonalization disorder?	No, episodes must be recurrent
What is the treatment for depersonalization disorder?	Symptomatic treatment of the anxiety and depression associated with the episodes

IMPULSE CONTROL DISORDERS

How can impulse control disorders be characterized?	By an inability to resist harmful behaviors
What is intermittent explosive disorder?	Failure to resist inappropriately intense aggressive impulses that lead to assault or damage of property
What is the treatment for intermittent explosive disorder?	SSRIs, antiepileptics, propranolol, and lithium have all shown effectiveness, as has group therapy. But there is no definitive treatment for this disorder.
What is kleptomania?	Failure to resist urges to steal objects that are not "needed" by the patient, with an accompanying pleasurable feeling
Are symptoms more pronounced during stressful times?	Yes

What other psychiatric disorder is commonly associated with kleptomania?	Bulimia nervosa: Approximately 25% of all bulimics exhibit signs of kleptomania. Other disorders associated with kleptomania include mood disorders, anxiety disorders, and substance abuse.
What is the treatment for kleptomania?	Therapy (insight-oriented or behavioral) and SSRIs
What is pyromania?	Recurrent episodes of intentional fire setting
What is trichotillomania?	Recurrent pulling out of one's hair (usually scalp) resulting in disfiguring hair loss. The act relieves tension that is present before the hair pulling. It is believed to be related to obsessive-compulsive disorder (OCD).
What is the treatment for trichotillomania?	SSRIs, antipsychotics, lithium, hypnosis, behavioral therapy, and relaxation techniques have all been used.

CLINICAL VIGNETTES

A 24-year-old woman is seen by her OB-GYN, and during the pelvic examination the doctor is unable to pass her finger into the patient's vagina. The woman says that her husband has noticed this lately during intercourse. The OB-GYN suspects that the woman has vaginismus. What is a treatment option for the woman?

Desensitization; the treatment for vaginismus centers on desensitizing the woman to penetration. In an intimate situation with her husband, they can try to desensitize her with light vaginal touching. As she becomes more comfortable, they can initiate more sexually exciting touching until penetration can be achieved.

A 45-year-old man and his wife are seeing a doctor to try to obtain "Viagra" for his erectile dysfunction. While taking the man's history, the doctor learns that he does have erections while sleeping (according to the wife) but is unable to obtain an erection prior to attempted sexual intercourse. Given this piece of information, what is the most likely etiology of the man's erectile dysfunction?

Psychological causes; if the patient is able to have an erection during sleep, then the cause of his erectile dysfunction is unlikely to be organic. Viagra can be prescribed for men with erectile dysfunction due to psychological causes.

A 31-year-old man is arrested after a woman complains that he was rubbing his genitals against her leg on the subway. When interviewed by police, the man claims he is seeking help from a psychiatrist for a disorder. What is he likely being treated for?

Frotteurism; frotteurism is sexual excitement derived from rubbing one's genitals on unsuspecting people, usually in a crowded place.

A 23-year-old man discusses his sexual life with his psychiatrist. He talks about his upbringing, which he describes as nothing out of the ordinary. His parents bought him toy soldiers and toy power tools. He never played with his sister's dolls. He was pushed to play sports and enlisted in the military at age 18. He had good relationships with his family and identified with his father. After leaving the military at age 21 he began to associate with a new crowd of friends. Often times he dresses as a female when he socializes but dresses as a man for work. He is not interested in undergoing surgical procedures to alter his genitals. He is attracted to other men and currently is satisfied with his relationship with another man. How can this person be described in terms of gender identity, gender role, and sexual identity?

Male gender identity, female gender role when socializing, homosexual sexual identity; gender identity refers to a somewhat permanent sense of being male or female as determined by upbringing. This identity is generally established by age 3. This person's gender identity is male. Gender role refers to a temporary or transitory affiliation of behaviors, attitudes, or dress associated with being male or female. Although most of the time this person dresses male, his gender role can be described as female when he socializes. Sexual identity refers to preference in gender for sexual relations as determined by the individual. This person prefers males in his sexual relations; thus, his sexual identity is homosexual. In contrast to this example, it should be noted that most transvestites are heterosexual and most homosexuals do not cross-dress.

A 23-year-old woman complains that she has difficulty working at her new job because she feels that she steps out of her body and watches herself work. The woman claims that this happens on a near weekly basis, and she becomes very scared that it will happen more often. What is the best treatment for this disorder?

Symptomatic treatment; the history is suggestive of depersonalization disorder. Treatment is symptomatic, and in this case SSRIs might be warranted to ameliorate the anxiety associated with this woman's episode.

A 28-year-old woman is involved in a car accident and is stuck inside her burning car before being rescued by firemen. She is hospitalized for minor injuries for 2 days and then released. In the following weeks, she experiences periods of time when she is overly focused on the car accident and times when she does not recall that it ever happened. When told about this dichotomy, the woman reportedly experiences panic attacks and is concerned that she is going crazy. What is the likely diagnosis?

Dissociative amnesia; she has impaired social functioning as a result of recurrent periods of amnesia related to a traumatic event. This meets the *DSM-IV* criteria for dissociative amnesia.

A 27-year-old woman is seen in clinic. She is sad and cries while explaining that she can't understand why her boyfriend left her. He told her that she seemed like "another person" on some days and was very inconsiderate to him. She can't recall acting like this. She gives her doctor permission to call her ex-boyfriend for more information, and her ex-boyfriend tells her physician how she would suddenly "change" into a mean-spirited woman who would inexplicably go out and spend inordinate amounts of money on clothes and jewelry. He says: "I always thought that she was bipolar or something." What is near the top of your differential diagnosis?

The differential diagnosis includes BD and dissociative identity disorder; it is unclear from the history if the woman truly assumed a different identity, but she does seem to fit that diagnosis, given her inability to recall the other identity and significant social impairment. More history, including drug use, mood symptoms, and medications, is needed to make the diagnosis. Furthermore, dissociative identity disorder is an extremely rare disorder.

CHAPTER 13

Law and Ethics in Psychiatry

PROFESSIONAL RESPONSIBILITIES

! What are the values commonly applied to medical ethics?

- Autonomy: the patient has the right to refuse or choose their treatment.
- Beneficence: a practitioner should act in the best interest of the patient.
- Non-malificence: "first, do no harm."
- Justice: concerns the distribution of scarce health resources, and the decision of who gets what treatment (fairness and equality).
- Dignity: the patient (and the person treating the patient) have the right to dignity.
- Truthfulness and honesty

What is confidentiality?

The long-standing principle that patients have the right to expect that information provided to a physician will be kept secret.

Is it acceptable for a psychiatrist to become personally involved with a patient after the termination of their doctor-patient relationship?

In their most recent code of ethics, the American Psychiatric Association (APA) unequivocally states that sexual activity with patients is a misuse and exploitation of the transference relationship, which may persist long after treatment ends.

What is euthanasia?

The administration of a lethal agent by another person to a patient for the purpose of relieving the patient's intolerable and incurable suffering. The American Medical Association's (AMA's) stance on this subject is that "[it] is fundamentally incompatible with the physician's role as healer, would be difficult or impossible to control, and would pose serious societal risks."

What is physician-assisted suicide?

The act of facilitating a patient's death by providing the necessary means and/or information to enable the patient to perform the life-ending act. The AMA's position is that this is fundamentally incompatible with the physician's role as healer.

! **In what situations can the confidentiality rule governing doctor-patient relationships be breached?**

1. Clinical information can be discussed among designated treatment personnel.
2. In the case of a subpoena, requested medical information must be released.
3. If **child abuse** is suspected, there is an obligation to report to the proper authorities.
4. A physician has a **duty to warn third parties of possible serious harm** to them by a patient if they are readily identifiable, and if the risk of harm is substantial and imminent.
5. During an **emergency,** essential information can be released.
6. If a patient is **suicidal,** the physician may need to admit the patient involuntarily and share information with medical staff.

! **What is the Tarasoff Duty?**

"Duty to warn": The obligation of a physician to inform third parties or authorities if a client poses a threat to himself or herself or to another identifiable individual. Specific guidelines vary by state.

What steps are health care professionals obligated to take in order to prevent a patient from committing suicide?

- Suicidal patients may be involuntarily detained for brief periods pending psychiatric evaluation.
- Reasonable steps such as close observation by nursing staff must be taken to prevent self-injury during treatment.

What rules govern the treatment and abandonment of patients?

1. Physicians have a duty to provide acute treatment during emergencies.
2. Physicians are not legally obligated to accept patients for non-emergent treatment.
3. Physicians cannot arbitrarily terminate treatment without providing the patient with treatment alternatives.

ADMISSION TO A PSYCHIATRIC HOSPITAL

! List and describe the two main categories of admission to a psychiatric hospital.

1. ***Voluntary admission***: Patient requests or agrees to be admitted to the psychiatric ward. The patient is first examined by a staff psychiatrist, who determines if he or she should be hospitalized.
2. ***Involuntary admission:*** Patient is found to be potentially harmful to self or others, so may be hospitalized against his or her will for a certain number of days. Each state has laws dictating the set number of days the patient may be hospitalized. After this period has passed, the case must be reviewed by an independent board to determine if continued hospitalization is indicated.

! What are some examples of potentially harmful behavior to self or others worthy of involuntary admission to a psychiatric hospital?

- Suicidal or homicidal behavior
- Inability to care for self

What elements of a patient's history are associated with an increased likelihood of violence?

- History of violence
- History of impulsivity
- Psychiatric diagnosis
- Specific threat with a plan
- Substance abuse

! What is the best predictor of future violence?

Previous history of violence

What must be provided to patients when they are involuntarily admitted to a psychiatric hospital?

Commitment or "hold" papers, explanation of their rights, opportunity to ask any question regarding their commitment

What are the rights of an individual committed involuntarily to a psychiatric hospital?

Patients who are admitted against their will retain legal rights and can contest their admission in court at any time.

What is parens patriae?

Legal doctrine that allows civil commitment for citizens unable to care for themselves

INFORMED CONSENT

What is informed consent?

The process by which patients knowingly and voluntarily agree to a treatment or procedure

! **List and describe the three components for informed consent.**

1. ***Information***: Patient must be informed of risks, benefits, and alternatives to the treatment.
2. ***Voluntariness***: Informed consent cannot be explicitly or implicitly coerced.
3. ***Capacity***: Patient must have the understanding and judgment necessary to make the decision.

! **What situations do not require informed consent?**

- Lifesaving medical emergency.
- Suicide or homicide prevention (involuntary hospitalization).
- Minors—Physicians must obtain consent from parents **except** when giving **obstetric care,** treatment for **sexually transmitted diseases (STDs),** or treatment for **substance abuse**. In these cases, consent may be obtained from the minor directly, and information must be kept confidential from parents.
- Therapeutic privilege—In rare circumstances, a physician may elect not to divulge information about a procedure to a patient because the information would be extremely harmful for the patient to know. The reasoning behind this decision must be carefully documented in the medical record.

What are "emancipated minors"?

Minors are emancipated if they:

- are self-supporting
- are in the military
- are married
- have children

What rules pertain to emancipated minors regarding informed consent?

Emancipated minors are considered competent to give consent for all medical care without input from their parents.

COMPETENCE AND CAPACITY

! What is the difference between "competence" and "capacity"?

Competence and capacity are terms that refer to a patient's ability to make informed treatment decisions. Competence is a legal term and can only be decided by a judge, whereas capacity is a clinical term and may be assessed by physicians.

! What criteria must a patient meet in order to be considered to have decisional capacity?

1. Understands the relevant information regarding treatment, such as purpose, risks, benefits, and alternatives
2. Appreciates the situation and its potential impact or consequences according to his or her own value system and understands the ramifications of refusing treatment
3. Can logically manipulate information regarding the situation and reach rational conclusions
4. Expresses a clear choice or preference over time (ie, consistency)

How should a person designated as health care proxy make decisions for a patient who lacks decisional capacity?

Current legal approaches require health care proxy to make decisions based on the principle of **substituted judgment,** which means that the decision maker should try to make the decision based on what the patient would do if he or she could make decisions on his or her own. In the absence of any idea of what the patient might want, the decision maker should use the **best-interests approach,** which involves making the decision based on what could reasonably be expected to be the in the best interests of the patient in the situation at hand.

How can the physician determine if a patient understands information regarding treatment?

The patient must be able to explain this information to the physician.

What criteria must a patient meet in order to be considered competent to stand trial?

- Understand charges against him or her
- Have the ability to work with an attorney
- Understand consequences
- Be able to testify

MEDICAL MALPRACTICE

! What conditions must be met in order to prove that medical malpractice occurred?

1. *A duty was owed:* A legal duty exists whenever a hospital or health care provider undertakes care or treatment of a patient.
2. *A duty was breached:* The provider failed to conform to the relevant standard of care.
3. *Damages*: The deviation resulted in damages (monetary, physical, or emotional) to the patient.
4. *Direct causation*: The breach of duty was a proximate cause of the damages.

Think of the 4 Ds: Divergence from a **d**uty that **d**irectly caused **d**amages.

! What is the most frequent basis for malpractice claims brought against psychiatrists?

Improper treatment accounts for 33% of all malpractice claims against psychiatrists. Next are cases involving attempted or completed suicide, which account for 20% of all claims.

What principles can reduce the likelihood of malpractice and liability?

- Document all important clinical observations, actions, and reasons in the medical record.
- Seek consultation and document the opinions of colleagues in the medical record.
- Communicate clearly and effectively with patients and their families.

What are compensatory damages?

Awarded to patient as reimbursement for medical expenses, lost salary, or physical suffering

What are punitive damages?

Awarded to the patient only in order to "punish" the doctor for gross negligence or carelessness

FORENSIC PSYCHIATRY

A physician called as an expert witness is primarily responsible for what?

Medical expert witnesses are called to present their professional opinions based on reasonable medical certainty.

! **What is the modern standard for the insanity defense?**

American Law Institute test: holds that a person with a mental disease/defect should not be held criminally responsible if the person (1) could not appreciate the wrongfulness of the conduct and (2) could not conform the conduct to the requirements of the law.

! **What are examples of previous legal standards for the insanity defense that are no longer used?**

- "Wild beast" test (1724): An individual is not guilty if he/she is totally deprived of his/her understanding and memory and knew what he/she was doing "no more than a wild beast or a brute, or an infant."
- M'Naghten rule (1843): An individual is not guilty by reason of insanity if, as a result of a mental defect, the person did not know the nature of what he/she was doing or did not know that what he/she was doing was wrong.
- "Irresistible impulse" rule (1922): An individual is not responsible for a criminal act if he/she was unable to resist that act due to a mental illness.
- Durham rule (1954): An individual is not criminally responsible if his/her unlawful act was the **product** of a mental disease/defect. Also called the "**product test**."

What is required to demonstrate criminal responsibility?

1. Criminal intent (**mens rea,** or "guilty mind")
2. Criminal act (**actus reus**)

CLINICAL VIGNETTES

An 84-year-old woman selects her husband for medical decision making because she knows that her cognitive abilities will deteriorate due to a recent diagnosis of frontotemporal dementia. Two years later, the woman's disease has progressed to the point that she is not capable of making medical decisions for herself. Her physician recommends a new experimental drug that will increase levels of acetylcholine in her brain. How should the patient's husband make the decision of whether or not to have the medication administered?

Current legal approaches require health care proxy to make decisions based on the principle of **substituted judgment,** which means that the decision maker should try to make the decision based on what the patient would do if he or she could make decisions on his or her own. In the absence of any idea of what the patient might want, the decision maker should use the **best-interests approach,** which involves making the decision based on what could reasonably be expected to be the in the best interests of the patient in the situation at hand.

The family of a 49-year-old man with chronic schizophrenia brings a lawsuit against his psychiatrist after the man develops repeated grimacing and lip-smacking movements. The family is concerned that the man's antipsychotic medication may have caused these effects. On what grounds could a lawsuit such as this be successful?

The case could be successful if the psychiatrist failed to obtain adequate **informed consent** from the patient at the time of its initiation. The three necessary components of this discussion would have been **information** (risks, benefits, and alternatives were provided), **voluntariness** (consent could not have been coerced), and **capacity** (the patient must have had the understanding and judgment necessary to make the decision).

A 25-year-old man is brought to a psychiatrist by his girlfriend because he "has not been sleeping for the last week." On examination, the man displays several symptoms of mania, including pressured speech, distractibility, grandiosity, and flight of thought. The psychiatrist diagnoses the man with BD and prescribes 300 mg lithium bid. Later, the patient's insurance company requests the records of this patient's treatment. How should the physician respond?

The physician must obtain authorization from the patient in order to release his medical records. Insurance companies cannot compel psychiatrists to release patient records, although they can deny benefits if the records are not released.

A 37-year-old man brings a malpractice suit against his physician. He claims that his physician deviated from the standard of care in not prescribing him antihypertensive medication to treat his high blood pressure, which resulted in him having a heart attack. What must the patient's lawyer prove in order to show that malpractice occurred?

Think of the **4 D**s: The lawyer must prove that there was a **d**ivergence from the standard of care (**d**uty) that **d**irectly caused the patient's heart attack (**d**amages).

A 46-year-old man is in the final stages of prostate cancer and is being kept alive with life support measures. The cancer has metastasized, and the patient's physicians predict that his life expectancy is less than 6 months. The patient expresses a wish to have his life support removed. A psychiatric evaluation is performed, and the patient is found to be of sound mind and able to fully understand the consequences of his decision. However, his family members disagree with his decision and wish to go to court to keep him alive. What is the most appropriate next step of action?

Since the patient is competent, the life support should be withdrawn in accordance with his wishes.

A psychiatrist begins seeing a former patient intimately. Their romantic relationship began about 1 year after their therapeutic relationship ended. What are the relevant ethical and legal issues?

In its code of ethics, the American Psychiatric Association (APA) states that sexual activity with patients is unethical. Such activity is viewed as a misuse and exploitation of the transference relationship, which may persist long after treatment ends. Insurance carriers for the APA and the American Medical Association (AMA) exclude liability for any such sexual activity.

CHAPTER 14

Psychopharmacology

ANTIDEPRESSANTS

What is the mechanism of action for selective serotonin reuptake inhibitors (SSRIs)?

Increase level of serotonin in synapse by binding to presynaptic serotonin reuptake proteins so as to inhibit reuptake

What is the mechanism of action for serotonin-norepinephrine inhibitors (SNRIs)?

Block the reuptake of serotonin and norepinephrine

What is the mechanism of action for tricyclic antidepressants (TCAs)?

Block presynaptic uptake of both serotonin and norepinephrine

What is the mechanism of action for monoamine oxidase inhibitors (MAOIs)?

Inhibit the activity of monoamine oxidase, thus preventing the breakdown of monoamine neurotransmitters such as serotonin, epinephrine, and norepinephrine

! What are some advantages of using SS/NRIs over TCAs or MAOIs?

SS/NRIs have very low sedative, anticholinergic, and orthostatic properties, and they are safer in overdose. There is also no need to avoid tyramine in the diet as a patient taking an MAOI would.

! How long does it take for the antidepressant effects of SS/NRIs to appear?

4-6 weeks. Energy symptoms (such as psychomotor retardation) tend to improve before mood.

When do the adverse drug reactions to SS/NRIs become most apparent?

Within 1-2 weeks of initiating therapy. Clinicians should also reassess suicidal ideations during this time period.

! What are some common side effects of SS/NRIs?

- Sexual side effects such as decreased libido or delayed orgasm
- Gastrointestinal (GI) upset
- Headache
- Weight gain (tends to occur over months of treatment)

What is another side effect of SS/NRIs that can appear within the first few days of treatment?

Mild anxiety. It is important to advise patients that this is a common side effect and that it typically resolves within the first week or two of treatment.

What are some ways to treat the sexual side effects of SS/NRIs?

- Add Viagra or bupropion (Wellbutrin)
- Reduce dosage (sexual side effects are dose-dependent)
- Advise patient to not take medication on day during which sexual activity is anticipated (ie, drug holiday). Note that this strategy must be balanced with the risks of discontinuation syndrome, decreased compliance, and recurrence of depressive symptoms.

What are some unique features of fluoxetine (Prozac)?

Its long half life (5 days) makes it an appropriate choice for patients with poor compliance and also decreases the risk of discontinuation syndrome. It is also somewhat more activating than other SSRIs and less likely to cause weight gain.

What are some unique features of citalopram (Celexa)?

It has the least drug-drug interactions of the antidepressants and is generally well-tolerated, making it a good choice in the elderly population or in other patients who are taking multiple medications.

What are some unique features of paroxetine (Paxil)?

It has a shorter half-life, is associated with anticholinergic side effects (such as sedation), is associated with weight gain more often than other SSRIs, and has numerous drug-drug interactions, making it often a less-than-ideal choice for treatment of depression.

In what instance can paroxetine (Paxil) be a good treatment choice?

Depressed patients with comorbid anxiety may benefit from its sedating side effect.

! **What is "SSRI discontinuation syndrome"?**

Most SS/NRIs—especially paroxetine (Paxil), venlafaxine (Effexor), and duloxetine (Cymbalta), which have relatively shorter half-lives—are associated with symptoms such as dizziness, electric shock-like sensations, sweating, gastrointestinal symptoms, insomnia, and general "flu-like" symptoms when discontinued immediately rather than tapered.

How is SSRI discontinuation syndrome treated?	Recommencing the original or lesser dose of the S/NSRI (or a similar S/NSRI), or slowly reducing the dosage over several weeks or months
What are some common SNRIs?	Venlafaxine (Effexor) and duloxetine (Cymbalta)
What is an advantage of venlafaxine (Effexor) and duloxetine (Cymbalta)?	In addition to depression, they can be used to treat pain secondary to neuropathy or fibromyalgia.
What is a unique side effect of venlafaxine (Effexor)?	Hypertension (worse at doses >225 mg)
In addition to depression, what else can SS/NRIs be used to treat?	Anxiety disorders (eg, panic disorder and OCD), some personality disorders, and eating disorders
What is trazodone, what is its mechanism of action, and what is used to treat?	It is an antidepressant of the serotonin antagonist and reuptake inhibitor class. In addition to depression, it is used in lower doses (50-100 mg) to treat insomnia.
! **What dangerous side effect is associated with trazodone?**	Priapism
! **In what populations should TCAs be avoided?**	Suicidal patients: TCAs are lethal in overdose.
Why should TCAs be avoided in the elderly?	**Orthostatic hypotension** may occur and put an elderly patient at an increased risk of falling. Elderly patients may be more sensitive to the **anticholinergic** side effects of a TCA such as dry mouth, constipation, urinary hesitancy, blurred near vision, confusion, delirium, and constipation.
Name another serious side effect of a TCA.	**Cardiotoxicity**. TCAs may cause cardiac arrhythmias, heart block, or prolongation of PR, QRS, and QT intervals. Patients with conduction system disease should avoid TCAs.
What is a common nonpsychiatric use of nortriptyline?	Used to treat chronic pain
What is clomipramine commonly used to treat in addition to depression?	OCD

! **What dietary changes must a patient make while taking an MAOI?**	Avoid tyramine-rich foods such as aged cheese; dried, aged, smoked, fermented fish and poultry; tap and unpasteurized beers; marmite and sauerkraut; and soy products and tofu.
! **What may result from taking MAOIs and ingesting foods rich in tyramine?**	Hypertensive crisis
! **What drugs, if used in combination with MAOIs, can cause a hypertensive crisis?**	Those that stimulate adrenergic receptors, such as decongenstants containing phenylephrine or oxymetazoline, stimulants (eg, amphetamines, methylphenidate), TCAs, SNRIs, and bupropion (Wellbutrin)
How is a hypertensive crisis treated?	• IV phentolamine • Continuous IV nitroprusside infusion
What are the main side effects of MAOIs?	Orthostatic hypotension, sedation
What are specific side effects of the MAOI phenelzine (Nardil)?	Sedation and weight gain
What is the mechanism of action of bupropion (Wellbutrin)?	Inhibiting the uptake of dopamine and norepinephrine
What is the major advantage of using bupropion (Wellbutrin) as compared to SSRIs?	Lower incidence of sexual side effects and weight gain
What are some disadvantages of using bupropion (Wellbutrin) compared to other antidepressants?	• At higher doses, bupropion (Wellbutrin) lowers the seizure threshold. • Bupropion (Wellbutrin) tends to be more activating and so may be less appropriate for patients who have symptoms of anxiety.
What is the mechanism of action of mirtazapine (Remeron)?	Modulates norepinephrine and serotonin
! **What are some unique features of mirtazapine (Remeron) that, in certain patients, can be advantageous?**	• Causes weight gain, which can be useful for patients who have decreased appetite or weight loss. • Low incidence of sexual side effects. • Causes sedation, which can be useful for patients who have insomnia. Less sedating at higher doses (ie, ≥15 mg).

Why must caution be used when using more than one antidepressant to treat depression?

Since most antidepressants increase serotonin, there is a chance of inducing "serotonin syndrome." Special care should be taken to prevent serotonin syndrome when starting an MAOI after a patient has been on an SSRI. Typically a period of 5 half-lives (~2-4 weeks) is used to "wash out" the previous antidepressant from a patient's bloodstream before starting an MAOI.

! **What are the signs/symptoms of serotonin syndrome?**

Symptom onset is usually rapid, often occurring within minutes:

- Cognitive: headache, **agitation,** hypomania, mental confusion, hallucinations, coma
- Autonomic: shivering, sweating, **hyperthermia, hypertension, tachycardia,** nausea, diarrhea
- Somatic: **myoclonus, hyperreflexia, tremor**

! **How is serotonin syndrome treated?**

Stopping the usage of the precipitating drugs, the administration of serotonin antagonists such as cyproheptadine, and supportive care including the control of agitation, the control of autonomic instability, and the control of hyperthermia. Those who ingest large doses serotonergic agents may benefit from gastrointestinal decontamination with activated charcoal if it can be administered within an hour of overdose. **Although if untreated serotonin syndrome can be fatal, upon the discontinuation of serotonergic drugs, most cases of serotonin syndrome resolve within 24 hours.**

! **Which are the best medications to use to augment the effect of SS/NRIs in treating depression?**

When used to augment SS/NRIs, atypical antipsychotics, mirtazapine (Remeron), and bupropion (Wellbutrin) have the most evidence in treating treatment-refractory depression. Lithium and thyroxine are also used to augment SS/NRIs but have less evidence of effectiveness.

MOOD STABILIZERS

What are mood stabilizers primarily used for?

Treatment and prophylaxis of manic episodes

What are some other less common uses for mood stabilizers?

- Potentiation of antidepressants and antipsychotics in treatment of depression and psychosis
- Enhancement of abstinence in treatment of alcoholism
- Treatment of aggression and impulsivity

List the most common mood stabilizers.

Lithium, valproate (Depacon), and carbamazepine (Tegretol) are the most common. Other anticonvulsants (eg, lamotrigine [Lamictal]) and atypical antipsychotics (eg, olanzapine [Zyprexa] and aripiprazole [Abilify]) are also effective.

What are the indications for lithium?

First-line treatment of acute mania and prophylaxis for manic and depressive episodes in bipolar disorder (BD). Also used to augment response to antidepressant therapy in depression.

What is notable about the therapeutic range of lithium?

It is very narrow (0.6-1.2); patients can become toxic at serum levels >1.5. Thus, close monitoring of patients' plasma levels is essential.

! What are the major side effects of lithium?

Fine tremor, sedation, ataxia, thirst, metallic taste, polyuria, edema, weight gain, cognitive effects (impaired learning and memory), GI problems, benign leukocytosis, thyroid enlargement, **hypothyroidism, renal damage, and nephrogenic diabetes insipidus**

! What lab tests should be monitored in patients taking lithium?

- Blood urea nitrogen (BUN)/creatinine
- Thyroid-stimulating hormone (TSH)
- ECG in patients >50 years or with history of heart disease, as lithium can depress sinoatrial node function

! What is the effect of lithium on pregnancy?

Associated with cardiac abnormalities (atrial-septal defects, eg, Ebstein's anomaly) and therefore is contraindicated in the first trimester of pregnancy. Women should receive a pregnancy test before starting lithium.

What factors increase lithium levels?	Nonsteroidal anti-inflammatory drugs (NSAIDs), thiazide diuretics, dehydration, salt deprivation, and impaired renal function
! What are signs/symptoms of lithium toxicity?	• Early: coarse tremor, nausea/vomiting, hyperreflexia, ataxia, T-wave flattening on ECG • Late: mental status changes, seizures, cerebellar dysfunction, coma
What are the psychiatric indications for valproate (Depacon)?	First-line agent for treatment of typical and mixed manic episodes and rapid-cycling BD
What aspects of BD is valproate (Depacon) better at treating?	There is some evidence that it is more effective for mixed states and rapid-cycling BD.
What is the mechanism of action of valproate (Depacon)?	Thought to increase central nervous system (CNS) levels of gamma-aminobutyric acid (GABA)
! What are the possible side effects of valproate (Depacon)? How should one monitor patients on this medication?	Sedation, weight gain, alopecia, GI distress, **hepatotoxicity, hemorrhagic pancreatitis, and thrombocytopenia**. Physicians should monitor a patient's liver function tests (LFTs) and complete blood count (CBC) regularly.
! What serum level of valproate (Depacon) is thought to be therapeutic?	50-100 mcg/mL
! Valproate (Depacon) use during pregnancy can lead to what side effect in the fetus?	Neural tube defects
What are the psychiatric indications for carbamazepine (Tegretol)?	First-line agent for treatment of typical and mixed manic episodes and rapid-cycling BD
What is the proposed mechanism of action of carbamazepine (Tegretol) for treatment of BD?	Blocks sodium channels and may also indirectly interact with GABA receptors
What are the side effects of carbamazepine (Tegretol)?	Skin rash, drowsiness, ataxia, pancytopenia, agranulocytosis, aplastic anemia, hyponatremia, and elevated liver enzymes. Physicians should monitor a patient's LFTs and CBC regularly.

What is the major cardiac side effect of carbamazepine (Tegretol) that can occur at therapeutic doses?	Decreased atrioventricular (AV) conduction. This may progress to AV block at toxic doses.
What is the overall effect of carbamazepine (Tegretol) on drug levels?	Strong enzyme inducer of the cytochrome P-450 system, so blood levels of carbamazepine (Tegretol) and other drugs may fall
What serum level of carbamazepine (Tegretol) is thought to be therapeutic?	4-12 mg/L
Lamotrigine (Lamictal) is generally used as an anticonvulsant, but is also used to treat what disorder?	BD, especially the depressive episode
! What life-threatening dermatologic side effect is associated with lamotrigine (Lamictal)?	Stevens-Johnson syndrome
During what phase of treatment with lamotrigine (Lamictal) does Stevens-Johnson syndrome generally emerge?	Almost all cases of Stevens-Johnson occur in the first 2-8 weeks of treatment or if the medication is suddenly stopped then restarted at the previous dose.
How is Stevens-Johnson syndrome associated with lamotrigine (Lamictal) treated?	At the first signs of rash, the medication should be held. If the rash abates, lamotrigine (Lamictal) can be restarted at the same dose and titrated slowly. If the rash progresses, immediate medical attention should be sought. It is estimated that 5% to 10% of patients on lamotrigine (Lamictal) will develop a rash, but that only one in a thousand patients will develop a serious rash.
What drug, if used together with lamotrigine (Lamictal), can increase risk for Stevens-Johnson syndrome?	Valproate (Depacon). It inhibits the metabolism of lamotrigine (Lamictal), causing higher serum levels and necessitating an even slower titration of lamotrigine (Lamictal).
What other medications can be used to treat bipolar disorder?	All atypical antipsychotics are approved for use in acute mania. Aripiprazole (Abilify) and olanzapine (Zyprexa) are also approved for maintenance treatment of bipolar disorder.

What medications are used to treat the depressive phase of bipolar disorder?

Lithium, lamotrigine (Lamictal), quetiapine (Seroquel), and fluoxetine-olanzapine combination (Symbyax) are approved to treat depression in bipolar disorder. Antidepressants are also added to mood stabilizers to treat depression, but they must be used with caution.

Which class of medications must be used with caution in patients suspected of having bipolar disorder, given their tendency to potentiate manic episodes?

Antidepressants

ANTIPSYCHOTICS

What are antipsychotics primarily used for?

Treatment of psychotic disorders, psychotic symptoms, psychomotor agitation, and certain movement disorders

What are the two classes of antipsychotics?

Typical and atypical antipsychotics

List some typical antipsychotics.

Chlorpromazine (Thorazine), thioridazine (Mellaril), trifluoperazine (Stelazine), haloperidol (Haldol)

List some atypical antipsychotics.

Risperidone (Risperdal), clozapine (Clozaril), olanzapine (Zyprexa), quetiapine (Seroquel), aripiprazole (Abilify), ziprasidone (Geodon)

! **What distinguishes high and low potency typical antipsychotics?**

- Low potency drugs—dosed in hundreds of milligrams, tend to be sedating, have strong anticholinergic properties, and are somewhat less likely to cause extrapyramidal symptoms (EPS). For example, thioridazine (Mellaril) and mesoridazine (Serentil).
- High potency drugs—dosed in milligrams and tens of milligrams, are less sedating, less anticholinergic, and more likely to cause EPS. For example, haloperidol (Haldol) and fluphenazine (Prolixin).

! How do typical and atypical antipsychotics differ in their side effect profile?

Atypical antipsychotics are associated with less risk for EPS and tardive dyskinesia. However, atypical antipsychotics can also cause EPS, especially, eg, risperidone (Risperdal) when it is used at higher doses (>6 mg). Atypicals are also associated with a higher risk for metabolic syndrome.

! Why must antipsychotics be used with caution in the elderly?

Both typical and atypical antipsychotics are associated with an increased risk for mortality in elderly patients treated for **dementia-related psychosis**.

! What are EPS, what drugs are they associated with, and how are they treated?

- *Dystonia*: Spasms of face, neck, and tongue. Occurs within hours to days and can be life threatening (eg, dystonia of diaphragm causing asphyxiation).
- *Parkinsonism*: Resting tremor, rigidity, bradykinesia. Occurs within days to weeks.
- *Akathisia*: Feeling of restlessness. Occurs after weeks.

EPS are associated with high potency typical antipsychotics. Treat with antiparkinsonian agents (eg, benztropine [Cogentin], amantadine [Symmetrel]) and Benadryl. Beta blockers and benzodiazepines are used to treat akathisia.

Which atypical antipsychotic is known to have the least risk of causing EPS?

Clozapine (Clozaril)

! Describe the other side effects of antipsychotics.

- Anticholinergic symptoms: Flushing, dry mouth, blurred vision, altered mental status, fever. **Think: "Red as a beet, dry as a bone, blind as a bat, mad as a hatter, and hot as a hare."** Associated with low potency typical antipsychotics and atypical antipsychotics. Treat symptoms individually.
- Antihistaminic effects: Sedation.
- Anti-alpha-adrenergic effects: Orthostatic hypotension, cardiac abnormalities, and sexual dysfunction. Associated with low potency typical antipsychotics and clozapine (Clozaril).

- Weight gain.
- Elevated liver enzymes.
- Lowered seizure threshold. Low potency typical antipsychotics are more likely to cause seizures than high potency.
- Tardive dyskinesia: Darting or writhing movements of face, tongue, and head; appears many months after beginning treatment. Associated with typical antipsychotics and more often seen in women. Treat by discontinuing offending agent and substituting an atypical antipsychotic such as clozapine (Clozaril); untreated cases may become permanent.
- Neuroleptic malignant syndrome: Confusion, high fever, elevated blood pressure (BP), tachycardia, "lead pipe" rigidity, sweating, and greatly elevated creatine phosphokinase (CPK) levels. **Twenty percent mortality rate**. Associated with all antipsychotics, but most often seen with typical high potency antipsychotics. Treat immediately by discontinuing offending agent and providing supportive care.
- **Metabolic syndrome:** Hypertension, insulin resistance, abdominal obesity, and dyslipidemia. Associated with atypical antipsychotics, especially clozapine (Clozaril) and olanzapine (Zyprexa). Consider switching to different antipsychotics, such as a typical antipsychotic with less risk of weight gain or aripiprazole (Abilify), in patients with significant weight gain.

! List the major movement side effects of antipsychotics in terms of their time course.

Rule of 4s: dystonia (~4 hours) < Parkinsonism (~ 4 days) < akathisia (~4 weeks) < tardive dyskinesia (~4 months/years)

! How do atypical and typical antipsychotics differ in their mechanism of action?

Atypical antipsychotics are selective in binding to mesolimbic dopamine sites, as opposed to typical antipsychotics, which bind to mesolimbic and nigrostriatal dopamine receptors equally. Atypical antipsychotics also bind to serotonin (5-HT2) receptors.

What is thought to be an adequate trial period of an antipsychotic medication?	Taking the minimum dosage for 4-6 weeks
! **Which antipsychotic is most effective in treating psychosis?**	Research has shown that clozapine (Clozaril) is the most effective antipsychotic medication for refractory schizophrenia. All other antipsychotics (typical and atypical) are thought to be equally effective in treating psychosis.
! **What is the potentially life-threatening side effect of clozapine?**	1%-2% incidence of agranulocytosis: patients must receive weekly blood draws for the first 6 months (if normal, thereafter every other week) to check CBC.
What are some other problematic effects of clozapine (Clozaril)?	Decreased seizure threshold (risk increases at >600 mg daily), tachycardia, myocarditis, sialorrhea (drooling), transient hyperthermia
Which antipsychotic is recommended for treating psychosis associated with Parkinson dementia?	Clozapine (Clozaril)
What are the neuroendocrine side effects of antipsychotics?	Prolactinemia, secondary to dopamine blockade. This can lead to osteoporosis in both sexes, gynecomastia in men, and amenorrhea and galactorrhea in women. Treat with amantadine (Symmetrel) or bromocriptine (Parlodel). Prolactinemia is most often associated with risperidone (Risperdal).
What is another side effect associated with risperidone (Risperdal)?	Tachycardia
What antipsychotic medication is associated with pigmentary retinopathy?	High-dose (>1000 mg/day) Thioridazine (Mellaril)
! **List the atypical antipsychotics in order of their tendency to cause weight gain, from greatest to least.**	Clozapine (Clozaril) > olanzapine (Zyprexa) > quetiapine (Seroquel) > risperidone (Risperdal) > ziprasidone (Geodon) > aripiprazole (Abilify)
What are some side effects common to clozapine (Clozaril), risperidone (Risperdal), olanzapine (Zyprexa), ziprasidone (Geodon), and quetiapine (Seroquel)?	Hypotension, sedation, and weight gain

What are some unique features of aripiprazole (Abilify)?

It causes the least weight gain of the antipsychotic medications and is more activating than the other atypicals, the latter of which often leads to akathisia.

Which atypical antipsychotic is known to be abused (often in the prison population)?

Quetiapine (Seroquel): referred to as "Quells"

Which antipsychotics are known to prolong the QTc interval and thus should be used with caution in patients with cardiac problems?

The IV form of haloperidol (Haldol) and ziprasidone (Geodon). Other antipsychotics cause only modest prolongation of QTc. In patients with long QTc intervals (>450 ms), consider switching to an antipsychotic with less risk of QTc prolongation and monitor with frequent ECGs.

Which antipsychotic drugs are available in injectable form?

Haloperidol (Haldol), perphenazine (Trilafon), chlorpromazine (Thorazine), olanzapine (Zyprexa), and ziprasidone (Geodon). Thus these medications may be used in the acute setting to treat an agitated patient.

! Which antipsychotic drugs are available in long-acting ("depot") injection form?

Haloperidol (Haldol Decanoate, q 2-4 weeks), fluphenazine (Prolixin Decanoate, q 1-2 weeks), risperidone (Risperdal Consta, q 2 weeks), and olanzapine (Zyprexa Relprevv, q 4 weeks). These can be used in non-compliant patients.

ANXIOLYTICS

What classes of medications are generally considered to be the first-line treatment for most anxiety disorders?

SSRIs and benzodiazepines

! Why are benzodiazepines considered safer than barbiturates?

Benzodiazepines lead to less respiratory depression in comparison with barbiturates.

Compare the mechanisms of action of benzodiazepines and barbiturates.

Benzodiazepines increase the frequency of opening of GABA channels (chloride permeable), whereas barbiturates increase the duration of GABA channel opening. **Think: "barbiturate" = increased duration.**

! Which benzodiazepines are short, intermediate, and long acting?	• *Short acting*: oxazepam (Serax), triazolam (Halcion) • *Intermediate acting*: alprazolam (Xanax), clonazepam (Klonopin), lorazepam (Ativan), temazepam (Restoril) • *Long acting*: chlordiazepoxide (Librium), diazepam (Valium), flurazepam (Dalmane)
What are the major side effects of benzodiazepines?	Drowsiness, slowed intellectual function, reduced coordination, and risk for tolerance and addiction. Care should be taken not to combine benzodiazepines with alcohol as respiratory depression may ensue.
! What medication is used to treat benzodiazepine overdose?	Flumazenil
! What three benzodiazepines are safe to use in patients with liver failure?	**L**orazepam (Ativan), **O**xazepam (Serax), and **T**emazepam (Restoril) are all safe to use in liver failure as their metabolism does not require an oxidation step. • **Think:** "Patients who drink a **LOT** of alcohol should get: **L**orazepam, **O**xazepam, **T**emazepam."
! Which benzodiazepines are most commonly used to treat anxiety?	In the outpatient setting, clonazepam (Klonopin) and lorazepam (Ativan) are most often used. They are preferred to alprazolam (Xanax) due to their longer half-lives and causing less feeling of "reward," making them less likely to be abused. Diazepam (Valium) is also used less often, due to causing more feeling of "reward" and higher potential for abuse.
What are the nonbenzodiazepine sedatives that also work at the GABA receptor?	Zolpidem (Ambien) and zaleplon (Sonata). These medications exert the same effect as benzodiazepines but are from a different class of medication. They cause less physiologic dependence than the benzodiazepines.
What nonbenzodiazepine sedatives are best for sleep induction?	Zolpidem (Ambien), zaleplon (Sonata)

What nonbenzodiazepine sedative is best for sleep maintenance?

Eszopiclone (Lunesta), since it has a longer half-life

What is buspirone (BuSpar)?

This nonbenzodiazepine anxiolytic acts at the 5-HT-l A receptor but has a slower onset of action than the benzodiazepines. It is useful in alcoholics as it does not exhibit cross-tolerance with alcohol and has a low potential for addiction.

PSYCHOSTIMULANTS

What is the mechanism of action of methylphenidate (Ritalin)?

Stimulates CNS activity; blocks reuptake and increases release of norepinephrine and dopamine in extraneuronal space

What medications are used to treat ADHD?

Methylphenidate (Ritalin), dextroamphetamine (Adderall), and atomoxetine (Strattera)

What are some unique features of atomoxetine (Strattera)?

It has a long titration time (meaning that it takes weeks of regular use before it will take effect) and does not produce strong stimulating effects like most other ADHD medications, giving it a theoretical lower potential for abuse. However, it is known to be less effective in treating ADHD than methylphenidate (Ritalin) and dextroamphetamine (Adderall).

! What side effects are associated with the use of psychostimulants in children?

- Loss of appetite and weight loss
- Deceleration of linear growth (adult height not affected)
- Irritability
- Headaches
- Abdominal pain
- Crying spells
- Tics (rare)

What adverse effect prevents the common usage of the psychostimulant pemoline (Cylert)?

Hepatotoxicity

DRUGS USED IN ALZHEIMER DEMENTIA

What are the two most common classes of drugs used to enhance cognition in Alzheimer disease?

1. Acetylcholinesterase inhibitors
2. NMDA (*N*-methyl-D-aspartic acid) receptor antagonists

List the most common acetylcholinesterase inhibitors.

Donepezil (Aricept), tacrine (Cognex), rivastigmine (Exelon), galantamine (Razadyne)

How are acetylcholinesterase inhibitors thought to enhance cognition?

Cognition is partly mediated by cholinergic neuron projections between the basal forebrain, cerebral cortex, and hippocampus. In Alzheimer disease, the loss of these cholinergic neurons hinders the cognitive pathway. By reversibly inhibiting the breakdown of acetylcholine, more of this neurotransmitter is available in the synaptic cleft of the surviving cholinergic neurons.

What are the side effects of acetylcholinesterase inhibitors?

Bradycardia, diarrhea, vomiting, abdominal pain, increased gastric acid secretion, and urinary retention

! **What are the indications for acetylcholinesterase inhibitors?**

Mild to moderate dementia (ie, MMSE score <22)

What adverse effect is specific for tacrine (Cognex)?

Elevations in serum transaminases

What is the theoretical mechanism of action for NMDA receptor antagonists?

To block the effects of glutamate, slow calcium influx, and prevent nerve damage

What is the most commonly used NMDA receptor antagonist?

Memantine (Namenda)

What are the side effects of memantine (Namenda)?

Fatigue, pain, elevated BP, dizziness, headache, constipation, confusion

! **What are the indications for memantine (Namenda)?**

Moderate to severe dementia (ie, MMSE score <16)

! **Do acetylcholinesterase inhibitors or memantine (Namenda) reverse dementia?**

No; evidence shows that these drugs have only a modest effect and may slow the progression of dementia.

CLINICAL VIGNETTES

A 76-year-old man complains to his doctor of extended, painful erections after beginning a new antidepressant medication. What drug is he likely taking?

Trazodone (Desyrel) and nefazodone (Serzone) can cause priapism (painful erections).

A 56-year-old woman recently diagnosed with depression complains of difficulty in achieving orgasm during sexual intercourse. Which antidepressant should be initiated to treat depression and which should be avoided?

Bupropion or mirtazapine. Avoid SS/NRIs; patients taking bupropion (Wellbutrin) or mirtazapine (Remeron) have a lower incidence of sexual side effects. SS/NRIs, as a class of antidepressants, have a higher incidence of sexual side effects and may be avoided in patients already experiencing sexual dysfunction if other antidepressant treatment options are available.

A 53-year-old man with a history of alcohol abuse and depression is hospitalized for malnutrition. He is cachectic on examination without any lymphadenopathy, constitutional signs, or strong family history of cancer. A complete neoplastic workup is negative. The patient insists that his appetite is very poor and he has had trouble gaining weight because of this. Which antidepressant may be most appropriate in this case?

Mirtazapine (Remeron); in addition to treating depression, mirtazapine (Remeron) has the advantage of causing weight gain for patients who have decreased appetite or weight loss.

A 24-year-old man was started on haloperidol 2 days ago for persistent hallucinations and delusions. Today he began having muscle spasms in his neck, which led to dyspnea and subsequent respiratory distress. His mother immediately took him to the ED, where the attending physician noted that his eyes were fixed in an upward gaze, and that he continually twisted his neck to the left side. What is the diagnosis and subsequent management?

Acute dystonia (brief or sustained muscle spasm) is treated with IM/IV anticholinergic medications (eg, Benadryl or benztropine [Cogentin]) or benzodiazepines and by stopping the haldol or other antipsychotic medication that precipitated the event. Although any muscle group may be involved, it most commonly affects facial muscles (eyes, jaw, tongue). Acute dystonia occurs within the first 3 days of treatment initiation and is associated with high potency agents. Maintaining airway patency is imperative.

A 53-year-old man with a history of hypertension, BD, and asthma presents to his physician with a "metallic" taste in his mouth. He has never experienced this taste before and nothing seems to extinguish it. The taste is not associated with any specific foods. On further questioning the patient reports modest weight gain. Considering this patient's past medical history, what could be a possible explanation for the taste?

Side effect of lithium; if this patient has been on long-term lithium treatment for BD, he may be experiencing one of its side effects, metallic taste. Other side effects of long-term lithium treatment include weight gain, acne, hypothyroidism, and polyuria.

A 46-year-old woman with a known history of depression is brought into the ER. She is comatose and intermittently convulsing. An ECG shows a long QT interval. What drug did she most likely take?

TCA such as amitriptyline or imipramine; remember the 3 Cs of TCA toxicity: Coma, Convulsions, and Cardiotoxicity.

A 67-year-old man is found by his wife on the floor. In the ED, his wife explains that his medications were recently changed, but she knows that he was taking phenelzine in the past. He is tachycardic, diaphoretic, and exhibiting myoclonic jerks with a BP of 192/105. What medication was likely added at his last doctor's visit?

SSRI; when an SSRI is combined with an MAOI, "serotonin syndrome" can result as in this patient's case. This syndrome presents with the classic triad of hyperthermia, rigidity, and labile blood pressure. Before adding another serotonergic agent to a patient's regimen, it is advisable to wait for some time (ie, a "wash-out" period, or 5 half-lives) in order to clear the previous agent from a patient's bloodstream.

An 8-year-old boy presents to his physician with loss of appetite, weight loss, and abdominal pain. One year ago, he was seen in the office because of inability to concentrate, distractibility, impulsive behavior, and poor academic performance. Since then he has been taking his prescription medication with great improvement in these symptoms. At follow-up, the patient's blood is drawn and results are significant for aspartate aminotransferase (AST) = 94 and alanine aminotransferase (ALT) = 105. What medication is this boy most likely taking?

Pemoline (Cylert); pharmacologic treatment of ADHD includes psycho-stimulants such as methylphenidate (Ritalin), dextroamphetamine (Dexedrine), and pemoline (Cylert). Side effects of psychostimulants in children can include loss of appetite, weight loss, inhibited body growth, irritability, headaches, abdominal pain, crying spells, and rarely tics. Pemoline (Cylert) is not first-line treatment for ADHD due to its specific side effect of hepatotoxicity.

You are seeing a 30-year-old woman with a history major depression who is being treated with paroxetine (Paxil) 40 mg daily. She has been stable on this dose for years without a recurrence of depressive symptoms, and you have considered tapering her off this medication. She calls you one day at the office and tells you that she feels like she has the flu but "different." She describes body ache, gastrointestinal symptoms, and periodic strange sensations she describes as "brain zaps." What should you suspect?

SS/NRI discontinuation syndrome. Paroxetine (Paxil), venlafaxine (Effexor), and duloxetine (Cymbalta) have relatively shorter half-lives and are associated with symptoms such as dizziness, electric shock-like sensations, sweating, gastrointestinal symptoms, insomnia, and general "flu-like" symptoms when discontinued immediately rather than tapered. Discontinuation syndrome is treated by recommencing the original or lesser dose of the SS/NRI (or a similar SS/NRI), or slowly reducing the dosage over several weeks or months.

You are treating a 39-year-old man with a history of major depression with citalopram (Celexa) 40 mg daily. You recently increased the dose from 20 to 40 mg and the patient experienced a significant improvement in his depressive symptoms. However, he reports that at the same time, he has lost interest in sex. What is happening and how can it be treated?

The patient is likely suffering from SSRI sexual side effects. Such side effects are common, tend to be dose dependent, and include decreased libido, anorgasmia, and difficulty achieving an erection. Treatment strategies include decreasing the dose, not taking the medication on the day of sexual activity, or adding Viagra or bupropion (Wellbutrin) as needed. Since this patient's depressive symptoms only responded to a higher dose of citalopram (Celexa) the latter two strategies would be indicated.

You have a 33-year-old woman patient who is being treated with valproate (Depakon) for bipolar disorder. During your appointment with her she tells you that she and her husband are trying to have a child. She wonders if she should stay on her mood stabilizer. How should you respond?

This is a complicated question that requires a detailed conversation. You should advise her that the risks of staying on valproate (Depakon) are that it can cause neural tube defects in a fetus. At the same time, being untreated for bipolar disorder carries its own risks, and you must advise her of that as well. Depending on what medications she has tried in the past and her overall clinical status, you could suggest switching to another mood stabilizer with less risks in pregnancy. Finally, in spite of these risks, many patients do make the valid, informed decision to stay on their current mood stabilizer because they would rather not take the risk of having a manic episode during pregnancy.

You are treating a 37-year-old woman with a history of bipolar disorder with lithium 900 mg bid. She has been well-maintained on this dose without any manic episodes for 1 year, and her lithium serum level one month ago was 1.0. She calls you one day at the office and reports that she has noticed a tremor in her right hand. She tells you that she has been seeing a chiropractor recently for lower back pain and asks if this could have anything to do with it. What should you suspect?

Lithium toxicity. One of the first signs of lithium toxicity is a tremor. This patient may be taking NSAIDs for her back pain, and NSAIDs can cause lithium serum levels to rise. Thiazide diuretics, dehydration, salt deprivation, and impaired renal function can also cause lithium levels to rise. The therapeutic serum level range of lithium is 0.6-1.2.

A 59-year-old man with schizophrenia is hospitalized for community-acquired pneumonia. The patient's medical history is unknown but he states that he takes ziprasidone (Geodon) for his schizophrenia. He becomes agitated on the night of his admission and receives haloperidol (Haldol) 2 mg IV on three separate occasions over the course of 12 hours. The next day, he develops a ventricular arrhythmia which is diagnosed as Torsades de pointes. What is the cause of his arrhythmia?

QTc prolongation likely secondary to antipsychotic medications. Of all antipsychotics, IV haloperidol (Haldol) and (ziprasidone) Geodon are known to prolong the QT interval to the greatest extent. In patients with long QTc intervals (>450 ms) or a cardiac history, consider switching to an antipsychotic with less risk of QTc prolongation and monitor with frequent ECGs.

A 45-year-old man sees you for treatment of major depression. You start fluoxetine (Prozac) at 20 mg daily and ask him to follow up in 2 weeks time. At his next visit with you, he reports that he has not felt much improvement. What should be your next step?

Do not change therapy at this time. Antidepressants take 4-6 weeks to have a significant effect on the symptoms of depression. Even though this is the lowest starting dose of fluoxetine (Prozac), you should wait at least another 2 weeks before increasing the dosage.

A 21-year-old woman presents to you for pharmacologic treatment of major depression. She has never taken an antidepressant before. You suggest citalopram (Celexa) and start 20 mg daily. She calls you in a few days and tells you that she feels "really jumpy" and can't sleep at night, and that she has stopped taking the medication. What happened and how could it have been prevented?

Mild anxiety secondary to SSRI initiation. It is important to advise patients that this is a common initial side effect of SSRIs and that it typically resolves within the first week or two of treatment. This will prevent them from believing that they are having an atypical reaction and stopping the medication. One way to address this issue is to provide a low-dose benzodiazepine to be taken on an as-needed basis during the first few weeks of treatment with an SSRI.

A 45-year-old homeless man with chronic schizophrenia is seen in a free mental health clinic. He has had schizophrenia for 20 years but has always refused to take medications regularly. What is a good treatment strategy for patients who are noncompliant with their medications?

The physician can consider administering a depot injection; injectable depot injections such as haloperidol (Haldol Decanoate), fluphenazine (Prolixin Decanoate), risperidone (Risperdal Consta), and olanzapine (Zyprexa Relprevv) are effective in decreasing the rate of relapse in patients who are not compliant with daily oral medication.

A 52-year-old man with chronic schizophrenia visits his psychiatrist for a routine appointment. His psychiatrist notices that the man continually smacks his lips and grimaces. During the interview, the man blinks constantly, and his tongue occasionally darts out of his mouth. What is the diagnosis and subsequent management?

Tardive dyskinesia; switch to atypical antipsychotic or reduce current dosage; tardive dyskinesia is a late-onset of choreoathetotic movements of the tongue, face, neck, trunk, or limbs, associated with prolonged exposure to antipsychotic medications, especially typical antipsychotics. Patients can be managed by switching from a typical to an atypical antipsychotic, especially clozapine (Clozaril), which has the lowest risk for tardive dyskinesia, or by reducing their current dosage. Symptoms of tardive dyskinesia may persist despite treatment.

A 47-year-old woman with chronic schizophrenia is brought to the ER by her sister after she was found unresponsive with T 102°F. Her BP is 150/80, HR 120. On examination, she is diaphoretic, and her muscles are completely rigid. What is the diagnosis and subsequent management?

Neuroleptic malignant syndrome (NMS); discontinue offending agent (in this case from the anti-psychotic medication). This is a life-threatening neurologic emergency. NMS typically presents with confusion, high fever, elevated BP, tachycardia, "lead pipe" rigidity, sweating, and greatly elevated creatine phosphokinase (CPK) levels. The most important step in management is to discontinue the offending agent. Although their efficacy has not been confirmed by clinical trials, dopamine agonists such as dantrolene and bromocriptine have been used. NMS is associated with all typical antipsychotics. It is thought to be more rare with atypical antipsychotics.

Index